Oral Infections and Systemic Diseases

Oral Infections and Systemic Diseases:

Scientific Evidence from an Epidemiologic Perspective

By

Lise Lund Håheim

Cambridge
Scholars
Publishing

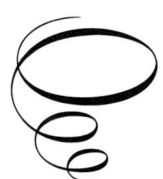

Oral Infections and Systemic Diseases:
Scientific Evidence from an Epidemiologic Perspective

By Lise Lund Håheim

This book first published 2022

Cambridge Scholars Publishing

Lady Stephenson Library, Newcastle upon Tyne, NE6 2PA, UK

British Library Cataloguing in Publication Data
A catalogue record for this book is available from the British Library

Copyright © 2022 by Lise Lund Håheim

ISBN (10): 1-5275-7735-X
ISBN (13): 978-1-5275-7735-0

TABLE OF CONTENTS

Part 3: Oral signs and symptoms of systemic diseases

Part 4: Cardiovascular disease research

PREFACE

A dentist is obliged to ask patients about their medical and dental anamnestic history of past and current diseases, medicine use, former dental treatment, and current oral health problems. That there may be a linkage between oral health and systemic disease has been considered by several researchers over the years, including the interest in infections being a cause of myocardial infarction.

Several conditions have been studied regarding a link to oral infections from a causal perspective. Diseases with some evidence of association with periodontal disease/periodontitis include cardiovascular diseases, cancer, diabetes, pneumonia, chronic obstructive lung disease, and pregnancy. More than 700 bacteria have been identified in the oral cavity, and this source of infection needs to be further explored. The main oral infections (such as gingivitis, periodontitis, and caries) have been thoroughly investigated and well described, and treatment options are available. However, little is known of their linkage to systemic disease. The aim of this book is to describe oral infections, such as dental and periodontal infections, and their consequences for general health using research information within the framework of the science of epidemiology. An epidemiologic approach is used to understand and explore the connection between health and disease, cause and disease outcome. The knowledge is built on studies of different designs providing evidence from different angles. The aim of this book is to provide an overview of the current scientific evidence.

To produce an updated knowledge of the scientific literature, subject items were searched systematically in PubMed. However, the number of scientific publications is large, and consequently, the risk remains that some publications known to others have not been identified and reported here. The focus was on recent literature from the last 20–30 years, as well as some well-known older publications to provide historic insight. The global interest in oral infections and systemic diseases among scientists has expanded greatly in the last 20–30 years. Initially, in the 19th century, infections were suggested to be related to and causal to heart disease. More recently, oral infections have been related to several diseases and conditions, and this book seeks to cover a range of these medical conditions. This knowledge may lead to improved understanding and preventive measures from a public health perspective.

It is fascinating to perform research in this field, as it associates oral health with systemic diseases. The importance of significant findings is of great value to improving an individual's health and public health from a wider public health perspective. Through this approach, I seek to explore the association between and causal aspects of oral infections and systemic diseases.

I am in debt and deeply grateful to Berit Mørland, Helle-Vibeke Wetterstad, Dag S Thelle, and Eiliv Lund for reading specific chapters and giving me their most valuable comments from their different professional positions. I am most grateful to my husband – Birger Håheim, who read the chapters and offered his comments to make the text more readable (as this is not his subject).

This book connects several research fields. The combined and broad scientific knowledge here is needed to understand if and how oral infections are associated or causal to different systemic diseases.

I hope this book inspires the reader.

Lise Lund Håheim
University of Oslo, Norway

PART 1:

SCIENTIFIC PERSPECTIVES IN ORAL HEALTH RESEARCH

CHAPTER 1

THE EPIDEMIOLOGIC PERSPECTIVE

Epidemiologic research is to build stone upon stone –
evidence upon evidence

Epidemiology provides a methodological framework to advance research in search of explanations and an understanding of the causes and extent of diseases. Studying oral infections and systemic disease is no exception. The aim is to better understand and support disease prevention and strengthen public health knowledge. This scientific knowledge is the basis for health promotion for the individual, as well as at the group and population levels.

Epidemiologic research includes a descriptive phase and an analytic phase. Studies have to be performed to collect data on individuals and populations and include several descriptive factors to untangle complicated questions on disease occurrence and consequence. It is clearly an area of research that includes different qualifications in medicine, dentistry, microbiology, statistics, or other fields. In-depth analyses and an understanding of often complicated biological processes are required, including bias analysis in study results.

The WHO website provides the established knowledge of oral health and what impact it makes on the world population (https://www.who.int/health-topics/oral-health/#tab=tab_1). The WHO state in May 2021, 'Oral health is a key indicator of overall health, well-being and quality of life'. (https://www.who.int/news/item/27-05-2021-world-health-assembly-resolution-paves-the-way-for-better-oral-health-care)

Oral health includes varied forms of diseases – for example, dental caries, periodontal infections (gum disease), other infections and autoimmune disorders, HIV symptoms, cancer, oro-dental trauma, noma (cancrum oris), and birth defects such as cleft lip and palate. Many of these diseases can require extensive treatment over several years. Teeth are important for eating, speech, support of facial structures, and appearance. It is therefore disturbing to read that the assessment of the Global Burden of Disease Study

2017 estimated that, '3.5 billion people are affected by oral disease worldwide'. Cancers of the lip and oral cavity, as reported by the International Agency for Research on Cancer, are among, 'the top 15 most common cancers, and about 180,000 die from oral cancer annually'. Further, the WHO acknowledge that, 'oral diseases and conditions share common risk factors with other diseases (noncommunicable diseases, including cardiovascular diseases [CVDs], cancer, diabetes, and chronic respiratory diseases)'. The WHO focus on three main factors to fight against – namely, 'tobacco use, high sugar intake and alcohol abuse – and claim diabetes is linked to the development of periodontitis progression. A causal link has been found between high sugar consumption and diabetes, obesity, and dental caries'.

More details about oral health can be found on the WHO fact sheet (https://www.who.int/news-room/fact-sheets/detail/oral-health). The importance of good oral health is obvious, as the WHO rightfully claims that, 'oral disease is a major health burden due to pain, discomfort, disfigurement, and even death. Tooth decay/caries is the most common health condition, and about 530 million children suffer from caries in their primary teeth. Adults suffer not infrequently from infection in the supporting tissues of the teeth, which may be the reason for tooth extraction'. The positive situation is that oral infections, to a great degree, are preventable and treatable in the early development of disease progression.

Why is the oral microbiome important, and what are its health functions? Deo and Deshmukh state that the oral microbiome plays a crucial role in maintaining oral homeostasis, protecting the oral cavity, and preventing disease development (1). They further summarize the functions of the different human biomes as follows: 'The microbial communities present in the human body play a role in critical, physiological, metabolic, and immunological functions, which include digestion of food and nutrition; generation of energy, differentiation and maturation of the host mucosa and its immune system; control of fat storage and metabolic regulation; processing and detoxification of environmental chemicals; barrier function of skin and mucosa; maintenance of the immune system and the balance between pro-inflammatory and anti-inflammatory processes; promoting microorganisms (colonization resistance) and prevention of invasion and growth of disease'.

Oral health matters to general health, as well as a healthy dentition and the oral cavity in general. The fact that oral infections and dental health affect general health has been discussed over the years. As dental diseases are common in the world population, associations with systemic diseases are of great importance. The degree of causality is more demanding to establish, but oral infections have been found to be linked to increased morbidity and to predicting mortality, which is of concern to the health service and public health efforts for populations. These associations include systemic diseases such as CVD, cancer, pregnancy, respiratory diseases, diabetes, rheumatoid arthritis (RA), and increased all-cause mortality. Other diseases will also be presented and discussed.

The relation between these different diseases may be due to infections where different factors are of importance, and not all have been clarified. Bacteraemia includes the spread of endotoxins, cytokines, and other products of bacterial activity during the infection process directly or indirectly, and the immune system responds accordingly (2). Oral microbiology is a complex subject. It is important to apply high-quality studies, and relevant covariates need to be considered, measured, and adjusted for in statistical analyses.

Humans need healthy teeth and gums for eating, speaking, the presentation of a smile, and well-functioning supporting structures of the head and neck. Bacterial infection either in the gum or as tooth decay are the main sources of bacterial infectious diseases of the mouth. In addition to an individual's immunologic response, research have shown that daily prophylactic measures are important to contain periodontal disease (PD) and caries. The control of tooth decay and healthy gums require daily cleaning of the teeth, sensible nutrition and eating habits, and fluoride to strengthen the enamel.

This book uses an epidemiologic approach to understanding associations between oral health and systemic diseases, including disease causes. In epidemiology, scientific methodology is used to study how risk factors can cause a disease in the short and long term and explore the prevalence, incidence, and mortality of the disease in question, considering other factors of individual risk or population characteristics. Epidemiology includes the individual perspective to understanding diseases. It forms the scientific basis for public health work in disease prevention and provides the scientific basis for good healthcare work.

Oral health affects many functions, specific diseases, and even total mortality. An early overview was given in *Stones' Oral and Dental Diseases* (3). In the chapter "Chronic Oral Sepsis and Its Relation to Systemic Diseases, Focal Infection", the authors cover this aspect in a modest way –the evidence ranged from early observations to more tangible evidence. The author briefly discussed the extension of oral infection into the alimentary tract, as bacteria are swallowed all the time. It was expected that some survive the acidic environment of the stomach (normal pH 1.5– 3.5). Later research showed that the bacterium *Helicobacter pylori* indeed survives and causes stomach ulcers. A focal infection is a secondary infection that has its origin in other parts of the body. The bacteria and/or bacterial products may be transmitted in the bloodstream and/or by the lymphatics. At the time of Farmer and Lawton's book, concern had been raised and assessed for several conditions (including CVDs and RA), but less was known of diseases of the nervous system, skin, and kidneys and possibly diabetes mellitus (DM).

Bacteraemia has been associated with atherosclerosis, diabetes, endocarditis, preterm birth, and other systemic diseases (2, 4, 5). In 1998, the American Academy of Periodontology (AAP) wrote a position paper on the role of PD in systemic diseases (4). The systemic diseases were bacteraemia, infective endocarditis (IE), CVD and atherosclerosis, prosthetic device infection, DM, respiratory diseases, and adverse pregnancy outcomes. In 2000, Joshipura, Ritchie, and Douglass considered there was enough causal evidence for chronic PD and tooth loss with risk for CVD, bacterial endocarditis, pregnancy outcomes, and all-cause mortality (5). More recent studies, including systematic reviews (SRs) of similar studies of different populations, have demonstrated that oral bacteria are associated with CVDs, RA, Alzheimer's disease (AD) or cognitive impairment, respiratory disease, chronic kidney disease, obesity, metabolic syndrome, cancer, and total mortality (6). Kane elaborated on oral health and the impact on atherosclerotic disease, pulmonary disease, diabetes, pregnancy, birthweight, osteoporosis, and kidney disease (7).

Some systemic diseases have oral symptoms such as ulcerations. These are prone to secondary infections by oral bacteria. This is well known, and the infections need to be treated appropriately. As dentists often see their patients regularly for oral health examinations, they are in a position to observe and assist in the early diagnosis of these diseases in cooperation with medical doctors. These diseases may include severe conditions such as leukaemia, scurvy, and syphilis (8). Dahlén, Fiehn, Olsen, and Dahlgren investigated oral symptoms of anaemia, benign mucous membrane pemphigoid, pemphigus vulgaris, Crohn's disease, Addison's disease, Behçet's syndrome, HIV, thrombocytopenia, and leukaemia (2). Other systemic diseases may cause other signs and symptoms, such as swelling of the salivary glands, bone lesions, afflictions of the tongue, and cancers of distant origin. Extensive scientific literature can be found in standard textbooks, on PubMed, and on other relevant trusted sites. Many disorders have been associated with oral infections, and this review will examine the current evidence of these conditions in separate chapters.

In 1965, Bradford Hill discussed cause and effect using principles of epidemiological evidence (9). He defined nine conditions that need to be explored before concluding on causality:

a) Strength of the association
b) Consistency
c) Specificity
d) Temporal relationship
e) Biologic gradient
f) Plausibility
g) Coherence
h) Experiment
i) Analogy

These conditions have caused debate and are still of great value in discussing principles and evidence. Kenneth Rothman, amongst others, argued that temporality (cause precedes consequence) is the main element to be fulfilled in deciding whether a risk factor is causal (10). However, the other elements on this list are highly relevant in a discussion on causality.

Different methods of registration of oral health in studies have been used. Regarding tooth health, caries status and causes and number of tooth extractions are mapped. Restorative treatment may include a crown, bridge, implant, and partial or full denture. Periodontal status is measured by gingival bleeding, pocket depth, number of affected sites, periodontal surgery, and alveolar bone loss. These measurements require clinical examination, X-rays, and self-reported dental disease history. Humans have teeth from the early days of life – named deciduous teeth/primary dentition. Later, the permanent dentition develops and replaces the primary dentition, and all, some, or a few are kept throughout life. The diverse measurements used in this research complicate this field regarding the comparisons of studies and their results (more information is given in Chapter 2). Moreover, there are several covariates/confounding factors that influence study results, and it is important to have knowledge and include measurements of these factors. Several textbooks on epidemiology are available for further methodological studies (10–12).

Concluding remarks

Prospectively following a cohort of people exposed to risk factors and unexposed people for a substantial length of time provides important information on the prediction of risk factors for disease outcomes. Intervention studies/randomized controlled trials (RCTs) that prove disease reversal are important. Retrospective case-control studies can be used to study rare conditions or as preliminary studies, but they are sensitive to information bias.

The oral cavity is not an isolated entity of the body; it has a mutual relationship with different organs of the body. More research is needed, and this book provides some insight and an overview.

References

1.	Deo, PN, and Deshmukh, R. 2019. "Oral Microbiome: Unveiling the Fundamentals." *Journal of Oral and Maxillofacial Pathology*, No. 23: 122–128. https://doi.org/10.4103/jomfp.JOMFP_304_18
2.	Dahlén, G, Fiehn, N-E, Olsen, I, and Dahlgren, U. 2012. *Oral Microbiology and Immunology*. København: Munksgaard.
3.	Farmer and Lawton eds. 1966. *Stones' Oral and Dental Diseases*. 5th ed. Edinburgh: E. & S. Livingstone.
4.	Scannapieco, FA. 1998. "Position Paper of the American Academy of Periodontology: Periodontal Disease as a Potential Risk Factor for Systemic Diseases." *Journal of Periodontology*, No. 69: 841–850.
5.	Joshipura, K, Ritchie, C, and Douglass, C. 2000 "Strength of Evidence Linking Oral Conditions and Systemic Disease." *Compendium of Continuing Education in Dentistry Supplement*, No. 30: 12–23; quiz 65.
6.	Linden, GJ, and Herzberg, MC, and Working Group 4 of the Joint EFP/AAP Workshop. 2013. "Periodontitis and Systemic Diseases: A Record of Discussions of Working Group 4 of the Joint EFP/AAP Workshop on Periodontitis and Systemic Diseases." *Journal of Periodontology*, No. 84 (4 Suppl): S20–S23. https://doi.org/10.1902/jop.2013.1340020
7.	Kane, SF. 2017. "The Effects of Oral Health on Systemic Health." *General Dentistry*, No. 65 (6): 30–34.
8.	Tyldesley, WR. 1969. *Oral Diagnosis. Oxford (Pergamon Press Series on Dentistry, vol. 7, Oxford).*

9.   Hill, AB. 1965. "Environment and Disease: Association and Causation." *Proceedings of the Royal Society of Medicine*, No. 58: 295–300.

10.   Rothman, KJ. 2002. *Epidemiology: An Introduction*. New York, NY: Oxford University Press.

11.   Kleinbaum, DG, Kupper, LL, and Morgenstern, H. 1982. *Epidemiologic Research: Principles and Quantitative Methods*. New York, NY: Van Nostrand Reinhold.

12.   Thelle, DS. 2015. *Epidemiology: A Basis for Public Health and Disease Prevention*. Oslo: Gyldendal Akademisk.

CHAPTER 2

ORAL HEALTH AND DISEASE MEASUREMENTS

This book is about oral infections and systemic diseases, and it covers the metastatic spread of infections from the oral cavity. It is not a book on how gingivitis and PD develop or how caries lesions advance from early lesions to pulpitis. This is well described in the literature. The aim is to explore current knowledge of why, how, and with what consequence oral infections can spread to other organs in the body and develop diseases. Research to map the dynamics of infection spread has not been fully explored. As many research publications have shown, there is an association, and the microbiology of invading organisms and immunology of the host need to be further explored.

The different research studies that have been published are prospective cohort studies, case-control studies, RCTs, and observational studies, often including laboratory studies of biological materials from study participants. The studies have used different measurements and registrations of oral infections, including different populations as male, female, or both and of different socioeconomic statuses worldwide. SRs with meta-analyses are therefore an advantage in finding stable risk estimates, as there are often large variations between the populations of the included studies, how and which oral parameters are measured, the comparators of treatments reported, and the choice of outcome(s). In addition, in recent years, this field of research has expanded, and a great number of publications is available.

Self-report information

Self-report information is commonly collected in cross-sectional surveys, prospective cohort studies, case-control studies, and repeated examinations. The questions need to be in common, clear language, with obvious and clear-cut response categories. It is advisable to test the questionnaire on several people in advance to ensure that the language is clear and cannot be misunderstood and that the response categories are well defined and relevant. Response categories to graded responses can vary, and the Likert scale, with 1–5 or 1–10 categories that may have additional response categories as 'not relevant' or 'do not know', is commonly used. The extent of the use of dental and medical services and drug use can be included. The number of teeth and reason for extraction, the degree and level of periodontal infection, other diseases and symptoms, and possibly the history of disease development are frequent questions. Additionally, questions on pain, bleeding of the gums, and loose teeth are relevant. Other dental infections may be pulpitis or apical periodontitis with associated pain as a consequence of caries. Aetiologically, there is an overlap, partially between the number of extracted teeth and chronic periodontitis. Extractions can be seen as a proxy for chronic periodontitis. Tooth extraction categories can, for example, be sorted by PD, caries with pulpitis, trauma, and orthodontic treatment.

Examples of questions on PD status used in studies are presented below:

'Have you had teeth extracted? Give the reason for tooth extraction (periodontitis, caries with associated pulpitis, trauma, or orthodontic treatment) and the number of teeth extracted. Do you have periodontitis? Do you have single-tooth infection? Do you have an oral infection?' (1)

'Have you had periodontal disease with bone loss?' (2)

'Have you noticed that some of your own teeth have come loose or fallen out on their own?' (3)

'Has a dentist or dental hygienist ever told you that you have periodontal or gum disease?' (4)

'Have you had periodontal bone loss diagnosed by a physician?' (5)

'History of gum disease diagnosed by a dentist?' (6)

Clinical measurements

Clinical measurements range in severity, from gingival bleeding as an initial symptom occurring due to tooth brushing to tooth extractions and alveolar bone loss due to chronic infections of the jaw. Table 1 presents a list of several indices by periobasics.com (https://periobasics.com/gingival-and-periodontal-indices/). These indices have been developed over many years, and as studies cover many years, the indices are used to varying degrees in publications. Other indices include the depth of periodontal pockets after advancing periodontitis and the extent of bone loss around the teeth, measurements of loss of attachment level, radiographic confirmation of alveolar bone loss, and the start and duration of symptoms.

Table 1. An overview of oral measures used in clinical practice and research

Registered oral condition	Terms for exposure
Self-assessment	History of tooth loss
	Diagnosed periodontitis/gingivitis/caries
	X-ray
Number of teeth, clinical registration	Tooth loss total
	Cause as periodontitis,
	apical periodontitis, trauma,
	orthodontic treatment or
	other causes
	Decayed, missing, and filled teeth
Gingivitis	Gingival index score
	Bleeding on probing
	PMA index
Periodontitis	Russell's periodontal index
	Periodontal disease index
	Pocket depth – standardized probe used
	X-ray
Periimplantitis	Periodontal disease index
	Pocket depth – standardized probe used
Alveolar bone loss	X-ray
Oral hygiene level	Plaque registration
	Debris index
	Calculus index
	Oral hygiene index-simplified
	Quigley–Hein plaque index
Other oral infections	Current or history of infection

Tooth loss

The number of teeth lost is commonly recorded in research. Teeth extractions due to infections are mainly due to PD, or pulpitis with periapical spread of infection through the pulp cavity, through the apical foramen, and into the surrounding alveolar bone which supports the tooth. Other main reasons are trauma and orthodontic treatment. The degree of caries status and other oral infections may be included, depending on the research theme. Denture use (full or partial design) and implants may also be recorded, as they are becoming more common. Concerning single teeth, tooth extraction can be seen to be the end stage of an oral infection. Extraction results in a premature loss of part of the permanent dentition and may include advanced dental treatment to restore oral functions.

Gingivitis and periodontitis

Bacteria, if not cleared away, can expand into the gingival crevice, the area where the tooth surface and the gingiva meet, and start the detrimental process of gingivitis and, later, periodontitis (8). This oral biofilm is called dental plaque and may be soft and colourless or become hard, called calculus. The plaque may become acidic if the sugar content is high, and this can initiate caries. Plaque bacterial complexes have been defined as yellow, violet, green, orange, and red (8, 9). The red complex is especially associated with aggressive periodontitis, and the anaerobe bacteria involved are *Tannerella forsythia* (Tf), *Treponema denticola* (Td), and *Porphyromonas gingivalis* (Pg) (9).

Caries and periapical periodontitis

The caries process is started by bacteria, and *Streptococci mutans*, *lactobacilli*, and *actinomycetes* are the main ones (8). The bacteria present also differ between sites such as enamel fissures, root surfaces, and dentinal caries. As more modern technologies are being used, especially 16S rRNA-based molecular methods, the spectrum of bacteria involved in caries has become greater and more diverse (7). Bacteria ferment the sugar nutrient in the mouth – producing acid, lactic acid in particular, and causing an acidic environment whereby calcium in the tooth enamel is released. The critical balance of demineralization is at pH 5.5. Saliva possesses the ability of alkalinization, as its pH is above this level. Frequent consumption of food of high sugar content exposes the teeth to acid for longer periods of time during the day, leading to caries progressing faster. If left untreated, the caries process deepens into the pulp and can cause infection with intense pain, and the tooth becomes painful to bite with. A widening of the periodontal space and a periapical abscess may be seen on an X-ray, confirming the diagnosis. This is a different situation from periodontitis – as there is no space inside the tooth for the infection to expand, except out of the apex of the tooth and into the jawbone and therefore causing pain.

Oral bacteriology

Dental plaque

The oral cavity harbours a large number of bacterial species, with different properties and different growth requirements and other microorganisms (such as fungi, viruses, and protozoa) (7). They may be common residents of the oral microbiota or transient microbes. The resident bacteria prevent the growth of pathogens, as they all fight for space and nutrients. Medicines or different nutrients may interfere with the growth of the normal oral flora, and the pathogens may exhibit unique factors allowing them to grow. The bacteria have different properties, but facultative anaerobes and anaerobes are the most influential bacteria in periodontitis. The bacteria and nutrients constitute plaque that adheres to the teeth and gingiva. This exists in the form of a biofilm – plaque, which is a three-dimensional structure composed of bacteria in a matrix of biopolymers that are important for binding to the different surfaces in the oral cavity (8). This matrix mainly consists of polysaccharides but also contains proteins and nucleic acid from the bacteria. The biofilm matures with the addition of more bacteria and more substrate. The biofilm may break off, and new areas of biofilm may be established. In the mouth, calcium deposits in stable areas of the biofilm; this is termed calculus. Plaque and calculus need to be removed daily to avoid disease. A biofilm can also form on other surfaces and cause infection in other areas of the body and on instruments that need to be frequently changed, such as catheters.

The oral microbiome

The bacteria in the mouth constitute what is called the oral microbiome, and over 700 species have been identified (7). With modern technologies such as new genomic technologies, including next-generation sequencing and bioinformatic tools, more bacteria have been added to the list (10). Genetic analyses to identify bacterial components have significantly advanced microbiology. The component 16S rRNA consists of 1,500 nucleotides and is part of the 30S subunit of ribosomes. Sequences of the 16S rRNA gene are important, as they identify both cultivable and non-cultivable bacteria (7). The component 16S rRNA can be found in all bacteria. The laboratory procedures are, in short, as follows: 16S rRNA is isolated and then amplified by polymerase chain reaction (PCR). The presence of bacteria is identified by species-specific primers. Alternative techniques are DNA-DNA hybridization for cultivated bacteria and microarray based on 16S rRNA identified bacteria, cultivable or non-cultivable. Currently, the Human Oral Microbiome Database contains 619 taxa and 13 phyla of the oral microbiome.

The oral microbiome is an integrated part of the human microbiome, which also consists of microbiomes of the gut, skin, and lungs (11, 12). In addition to bacteria, other microorganisms (such as fungi, viruses, and protozoa) can be identified in the mouth. The different areas of the mouth have soft tissues and hard surfaces of teeth, and these provide different habitats for bacteria – which, in turn, implies that in some areas, aerobic species dominate but in others, facultative anaerobes or anaerobes are predominant. Some areas are exposed to much abrasion by the masticatory apparatus itself, muscle movement, and the tongue, especially when chewing food and during speech.

The oral microbiome has adapted to the different environments of the mouth. It is crucial in maintaining oral homeostasis, protecting the oral cavity from disease development, and maintaining general health (13). The oral microbiome is easily accessible for investigation and has been much studied. The advances from standard bacterial culture growth to modern genetic analyses have facilitated the identification of a vast number of bacteria (13). The oral microbiome is structured and categorized in a hierarchy of taxa: phylum (topmost) and then class, order, family, genus, and species. The oral microbiome has 12 phyla identified: *Firmicutes, Fusobacteria, Proteobacteria, Actinobacteria, Bacteroidetes, Chlamydiae, Chloroflexi, Spirochaetes, SR1, Synergistetes, Saccharibacteria,* and *Gracilibacteria* (13). Dahlén, Fiehn, Olsen, and Dahlgren listed the following main genera occurring in the mouth: *Streptococcus, Actinomyces, Lactobacillus, Porphyromonas, Prevotella, Fusobacterium, Treponema, Tannerella,* and *Capnocytophaga* (8). There are over 700 bacterial species in the oral cavity, the lowest level in this hierarchy (9). Oral diseases are due to infection by bacterial species. Genes can be transferred between bacteria, making them more resistant to antibiotics and producing increased virulence.

Bacterial species related to periodontitis have been grouped according to potential pathogenicity for serious and chronic infections. In the mouth, anaerobes constitute the bacteria that cause the development of infection by tissue destruction – progressing from the gingiva to the breakdown of periodontal fibres that anchor the teeth to the alveolar bone, the breakdown of alveolar bone, and eventually, the loss of teeth. Bacteria causing caries also, if untreated, spread to the pulp of the tooth, causing pulpitis, and progress to cause apical periodontitis and alveolar bone destruction, resulting in root canal treatment or tooth extraction.

In 1998, Mattila, Valtonen, Nieminen, and Asikainen wrote a review of the current knowledge of studies on infection and CVD (14). They described several studies on bacteria and viruses but concluded that causality had not been established. Since then, much research has been done to further explore this area within the field of epidemiology. Socransky, Haffajee, Cugini, Smith et al. described a group of anaerobic bacteria in the subgingival plaque found to be causative agents of aggressive chronic periodontitis and termed them the red complex (9). The agents were Tf, Td, and Pg, which are found in deep periodontal pockets adjacent to one or more roots of teeth. Such pockets gradually deepen unless treated. If untreated, the pockets enlarge, and the teeth become loose. Other bacterial complexes described are termed yellow, orange, green, and purple and are associated with periodontal health (8). The orange complex is also associated with the development of periodontitis and includes the bacteria *Fusobacterium nucleatum* (Fn), *Campylobacter*, and *Prevotella* species, including *Prevotella intermedia* (Pi). The initial infection on tooth surfaces starts with the yellow complex of oral *Streptococci* (*S. mitis, S. oralis*, and *S. sanguis*) and *Actinomyces* spp. – followed by the purple and green complexes, including *Eikenella* and *Capnocytophaga*.

Immunologic response to oral infection

It is well established that bacteria are in the oral cavity, always have been, but how do they function in health and disease? There are some basic and underlying mechanisms in the interplay between bacteria and the immune system (15). The metastatic spread of oral bacteria is due to acute or chronic infections in oral tissues. Bacteria may stimulate the immune system to produce antibodies. If this is deficient, then the bacteria metastasize more easily, and inflammation or infection occurs at distant sites in the body. Bacteria also produce toxins that spread locally and systemically. It is believed that these mechanisms are the reason for full or partial unwanted influence in other organs of the body (10).

One bacterium of the red complex – Pg – has been investigated for its part in developing chronic periodontitis and its possible role in several systemic diseases (16). Fiorillo, Cervino, Laino, D'Amico et al conducted an SR and concluded that Pg is involved in the onset of different systemic pathologies, including RA, cardiovascular pathologies, and neurodegenerative pathologies. The researchers sought a better understanding of the mechanisms of diffusion of this bacterium. In the red complex, there are two other bacteria – Tf and Td – and they benefit from each other to drive infection, causing tissue destruction. Håheim, Schwarze, Thelle, Nafstad et al. examined antibody levels to these three bacteria and *Actinomyces actinomycetemcomitans* and found that low antibody levels to Tf increases the risk of CVD mortality in men with a prior myocardial infarction (MI) (17). Immunological dysfunction of low levels of IgG antibodies, as observed, may be a reason for the spread of infection. This could be the missing link in the understanding of causal aspects of how chronic periodontitis can cause systemic diseases.

The involvement of other parts of the oral microbiome and the associated virulence capacity is of importance in the understanding of the link between oral infections and systemic diseases. Oral microbes, resident or invading ones, elicit an immunological response as a means of protecting the host, which eliminates the microbes, and exhibit cell-damaging properties (8). The microbes have properties to evade the host response. In the mouth, the microorganisms live in a biofilm of several microorganisms. For this reason, infections such as periodontitis and caries are chronic in nature and are more difficult to target and treat than acute infections of single microorganisms.

Serological measurements of inflammation and infection

The normal immune response has various ways of fighting invading bacterial pathogens. These include intracellular protection, inactivation, antibody production, inhibition of phagocytosis, inhibition of complement action, killing of inflammatory cells, or antigenic variation and mimicry.

Relevant bacterial products differ, and immunological response is graded between individuals. In microbiologic research, some common factors are analysed to understand the interaction between the oral microbiome and individuals in order to map causal pathways between infection and disease. Microbes may have cell- and tissue-destructive properties, such as toxins and enzymes. Toxins can be endotoxins or exotoxins. Lipopolysaccharide (LPS) is an endotoxin; lipid A is the main toxic part of the molecule and is released from Gram-negative bacteria. Pathogenic bacteria (bacteria able to initiate and cause disease) produce cell-damaging enzymes, including proteases as metalloproteases. Other cell-damaging enzyme categories are phospholipases, cytolysins, and streptodornase. High-sensitivity C-reactive protein (hs-CRP) is an acute-phase protein produced by the liver, is a serum marker of general inflammation in bacterial infections and cancer, and has been measured in many studies. Activated T-cells produce proinflammatory cytokines, such as interleukin (IL) 1, IL-2, IL-6, IL-10, interferon-γ (IFN-γ), and tumour necrosis factor (TNF).

Investigating antibodies to oral bacteria from the perspective of systemic diseases is uncommon, but a few studies have reported on levels of antibodies to PD and systemic diseases measured by enzyme-linked immunosorbent assay (ELISA) in search of a causal pathway from oral infection to systemic diseases such as CVD (17). Recorded levels may vary significantly. The presence of antibodies indicates that a person has had periodontal infection because the body has responded by forming antibodies. If the levels of some of these antibodies are low, it may indicate that infection has spread, as there is inadequate resistance by the T-cells of the immunologic system. This may indicate that some persons are more vulnerable to the spread of infection locally and systemically. This has been observed, and more research is needed to explore possible preventive measures, such as vaccination (17). RCTs using antibiotics to prevent heart disease could, in terms of this causal model, be too late, as the infection would have already spread to the circulation due to low levels of antibody production. Bacterial DNA has been identified in pathologic studies on aortic aneurysms (18).

Different systemic inflammatory reactions as hs-CRP, IL-6, and soluble E-selectin and immunological responses as IgG have been investigated. Intervention studies (RCTs) have shown that serologic measures related to inflammation are positively affected by treatment of PD (19, 20). Hs-CRP, IL-6, soluble E-selectin, and TNF-α have also been linked to CVD, obesity, and metabolic syndrome, and the lowering of elevated levels of these markers due to oral infection favours a better prognosis for these systemic diseases.

Concluding remarks

This chapter does not exhaust all issues in bacteriology and immunology of oral disease but provides some main lines for understanding and inspiration for further reading. There are many elements to explore to increase the understanding of these complex mechanisms in bacteriology and immunology. The factors mentioned show a great degree of potential heterogeneity when study results are compared. The heterogeneity is mirrored in potential risk factors investigated, a comparison of populations under study, interventions examined and comparators, and the consistency of outcomes between different studies. This is a challenge that needs to be considered when study results are compared and causality is discussed.

References

1.   Håheim, Lise L, Lund Larsen, PG, Søgaard, AJ, and Holme, I. 2006.
       "Risk Factors Associated with Body Mass Index Increase in Men at
       28 Years Follow-Up." *QJM*, No. 99 (10): 665–671.
2.   Arora, M, Weuve, J, Fall, K, Pedersen, NL, and Mucci, LA. 2010.
       "An Exploration of Shared Genetic Risk Factors between
       Periodontal Disease and Cancers: A Prospective Co-twin Study."
       American Journal of Epidemiology, No. 171 (2): 253–259.
       https://dx.doi.org/10.1093/aje/kwp340
3.   Mai, X, LaMonte, MJ, Hovey, KM, Nwizu, N, Freudenheim, JL,
       Tezal, M, Scannapieco, F, Hyland, A, Andrews, CA, Genco, RJ, and
       Wactawski-Wende, J. 2014. "History of Periodontal Disease
       Diagnosis and Lung Cancer Incidence in the Women's Health
       Initiative Observational Study." *Cancer Causes & Control*, No. 25
       (8): 1045–1053.
4.   Michaud, K, Pope, J, van de Laar, M, Curtis, JR, Kannowski, C,
       Mitchell, S, Bell, J, Workman, J, Paik, J, Cardoso, A, Taylor, PC.
       2020. "A Systematic Literature Review of Residual Symptoms and
       Unmet Need in Patients with Rheumatoid Arthritis." *Arthritis Care
       & Research (Hoboken)*. https://doi.org/10.1002/acr.24369
5.   Momen-Heravi, F, Babic, A, Tworoger, SS, Zhang, L, Wu, K, Smith-
       Warner, SA, Ogino, S, Chan, AT, Meyerhardt, J, Giovannucci, E,
       Fuchs, C, Cho, E, Michaud, DS, Stampfer, MJ, Yu, YH, Kim, D, and
       Zhang, X. 2017. "Periodontal Disease, Tooth Loss and Colorectal
       Cancer Risk: Results from the Nurses' Health Study." *International
       Journal of Cancer*, No. 140: 646–652.
       https://doi.org/10.1002/ijc.30486
6.   Mazul, AL, Taylor, JM, Divaris, K, Weissler, MC, Brennan, P,
       Anantharaman, D, Abedi-Ardekani, B, Olshan, AF, and Zevallos, JP.
       2017. "Oral Health and Human Papillomavirus-Associated Head and
       Neck Squamous Cell Carcinoma." *Cancer*, No. 123: 71–80.
       https://doi.org/10.1002/cncr.30312
7.   Aas, JA, Paster, BK, Stokes, LN, Olsen, I, and Dewhirst, FE. 2005.
       "Defining the Normal Bacterial Flora of the Oral Cavity." *Journal of
       Clinical Microbiology*. No. 43: 5721–5732.
       https://doi.org/10.1128/JCM.43.11.5721-5732.2005
8.   Dahlén, G, Fiehn, N-E, Olsen, I, and Dahlgren, U. 2012. *Oral
       Microbiology and Immunology*. København: Munksgaard.

9.   Socransky, SS, Haffajee, AD, Cugini, MA, Smith, C, and Kent Jr, RL. 1998. "Microbial Complexes in Subgingival Plaque." *Journal of Clinical Periodontology*, No. 25: 134–144.

10.   Kilian, M, Chapple, IL, Hannig, M, Marsh, PD, Meuric, V, Pedersen, AML, Tonetti, MS, Wade, WG, Zaura, E. 2016. "The Oral Microbiome – an Update for Oral Healthcare Professionals. *British Dental Journal*, No. 221: 657–666.

11.   Païssé, S, Valle, C, Servant, F, Courtney, M, Burcelin, R, Amar, J, and Lelouvier, B. 2016. "Comprehensive Description of Blood Microbiome from Healthy Donors Assessed by 16S Targeted Metagenomic Sequencing." *Transfusion*, No. 56 (5): 1138–1147.

12.   Castillo, DJ, Rifkin, RF, Cowan, DA, and Potgieter, M. 2019. "The Healthy Human Blood Microbiome: Fact or Fiction?" *Frontiers in Cellular and Infection Microbiology*, No. 9: 148.

13.   Deo, PN, and Deshmukh, R. 2019. "Oral Microbiome: Unveiling the Fundamentals." *Journal of Oral and Maxillofacial Pathology*, No. 23 (1): 122–128. https://doi.org/10.4103/jomfp.JOMFP_304_18

14.   Mattila, KJ, Valtonen, VV, Nieminen, MS, and Asikainen, S. 1998. "Role of Infection as a Risk Factor for Atherosclerosis, Myocardial Infarction, and Stroke." *Clinical Infectious Diseases*, No. 26: 719–734.

15.   Pedersen, AML. *Oral Infections and General Health: From Molecule to Chairside*. Springer, Switserland.

16.   Fiorillo, L, Cervino, G, Laino, L, D'Amico, C, Mauceri, R, Tozum, TF, Gaeta, M, and Cicciù, M. 2019. "*Porphyromonas gingivalis*, Periodontal and Systemic Implications: A Systematic Review." *Dentistry Journal (Basel)*, No. 7 (4): 114. https://doi.org/10.3390/dj7040114

17.   Håheim, Lise L, Schwarze, PF, Thelle, DS, Nafstad, P, Rønningen, KS, and Olsen, I. 2020. "Low Levels of Antibodies for the Oral Bacterium *Tannerella forsythia* Predict Cardiovascular Disease Mortality in Men with Myocardial Infarction: A Prospective Cohort Study." *Medical Hypotheses*, No. 138: 109575. https://doi.org/10.1016/j.mehy.2020.109575

18.   Marques da Silva, R, Caugant, DA, Lingaas, PS, Geiran, O, Tronstad, L, and Olsen, I. 2005. "Detection of *Actinobacillus actinomycetemcomitans* but Not Bacteria of the Red Complex in Aortic Aneurysms by Multiplex PCR." *Journal of Periodontology*, No. 76: 590–594.

19.   D'Aiuto, F, Nibali, L, Parkar, M, Suvan, J, Tonetti, MS. 2005. "Short-Term Effects of Intensive Periodontal Therapy on Serum

Inflammatory Markers and Cholesterol." *Journal of Dental Research*, No. 84: 269–273.
https://doi.org/10.1177/154405910508400312

20. Pussinen, PJ, Jauhiainen, M, Vilkuna-Rautiainen, T, Sundvall, J, Vesanen, M, Mattila, K, Palosuo, T, Alfthan, G, and Asikainen, S. 2004. "Periodontitis Decreases the Antiatherogenic Potency of High Density Lipoprotein." *Journal of Lipid Research*, No. 45 (1): 139–147. https://doi.org/10.1194/jlr.M300250-JLR200

CHAPTER 3

STUDY DESIGNS AND SYSTEMATIC LITERATURE SEARCH

Epidemiology is the scientific basis for good public health work. The field represents a systematic search for disease causes and is used to describe the extent of mortality, disease, and disease-related factors in the population. The aim is to contribute to disease prevention and improve public health. The major aims of epidemiologic studies are to study risk factors to help predict diseases forward in time, but sometimes retrospective data are found available and of interest. In epidemiology, it is a major task to map disease in any population and what factors influence disease prevalence, incidence, or mortality of selected disease outcomes. The temporal distance between measuring risk factor levels and outcomes is of major importance in having faith in study results and in that the results have not been influenced by any risk factors or other kinds of information. It is vital to have as little bias as possible in the recording of risk factors and known confounding factors and the results achieved. Information on outcomes can be found in hospital data, clinical registries, and mortality registries.

Following persons over time with regard to health factors provides valuable information. As science progresses, the scope of research changes with new scientific evidence, adding to the knowledge base for new health issues to be explored. One of the driving forces in CVD research after World War II was the rise in CVD prevalence, which caused great concern, and more information on treatment and prospective information was needed. Several approaches are applicable when exploring an association between oral disease/infection and systemic diseases. In earlier studies, the findings were sometimes accidental. In Mattila, Valtonen, Nieminen, and Asikainen's Finnish case-cohort study, oral infection was associated with MI (1). The study made a significant impact due to the novelty and quality of the evidence.

Epidemiologic research projects can broadly be described as being descriptive and analytic (2, 3). Before research starts, it is important to formulate a hypothesis and choose a study design. Common to all studies, it is important to map and reduce systematic errors in conducting a study. It is often of interest to describe the occurrence of disease and risk factor exposure. The aim can be to map health problems or plan health measures and to describe the characteristics of the actual population. Further analyses as comparing recorded risk factors relative to disease status, gender, age, geographical area, and so on to determine the prevalence or incidence of a disease – may follow.

Study designs

Below are tables presenting different study designs in a hierarchy with respect to the risk of bias in the results. This is especially important when studying the temporality of risk factors of disease or the effect of interventions. Study designs or modifications other than the ones listed here may be relevant to carry out the intended study. Each study design has its advantages and disadvantages, and the main study designs are listed in the following order: prospective cohort study (Table 1), case-control study (Table 2), case-cohort study (Table 3), RCT (Table 4), and cross-sectional study (Table 5).

Table 1. Prospective cohort study

Prospective cohort study
The basis is a health screening, a cross-sectional study where all factors of interest are recorded using a questionnaire, blood samples, body measures, or/and other measurements of interest. The participants are followed prospectively for the outcome of interest (incidence of or mortality from a certain disease). The cohort of individuals can, at a later date, have repeated measurements taken, or the data can be linked to outcome measures as registered in different registries or hospital records, for example. Person years of observation are also recorded.

Advantage	Disadvantage
Temporal analysis: It can identify patients with regard to disease or death in comparison to risk exposure	Limitations of which confounding factors are measured
Study the effect of risk factors by graded/dose response on the outcome	
Acquisition of follow-up data on incidence and mortality of disease	
Comparison of results between study groups	
Explanation of cause of disease, and mapping of causes in an etiologic context	
The registration of potential confounding factors is important for use in statistical analyses	

Table 2. Case-control study

Case-control study	
The cases are persons with a disease of interest to study. Often, these are clinical cases. In addition, one or more controls are selected. Both groups take part in a screening, and data is collected.	
Advantage	**Disadvantage**
The study of rare conditions/diseases	Recall bias of exposure and disease information
It is relatively cheap and simple to perform	Causality cannot be determined
Retrospective assembling of patient information	

Table 3. Case-cohort study

Case-cohort study/nested case-control study	
In an established prospective cohort, cases are selected (e.g. cases with a specific mortality diagnosis), and controls are drawn randomly.	
Advantage	**Disadvantage**
It can follow/identify participants with respect to disease or death through new data from sources such as disease registries, hospital data, or mortality statistics	It is dependent on which data and biological material were collected at the initial health survey
Data collection at the initial screening	
If biologic material was collected at the screening, this can be used for new analyses if permission is granted	
Testing of new disease hypotheses	
Limited systematic bias	

Table 4. Randomized controlled trial

Randomized controlled trial

A randomized controlled trial consists of two or more groups of randomized participants to study the effect of a treatment or intervention. The participants are randomized to be given active versus placebo or the best available treatment. The randomization procedure ensures the least biased assessment of the study results because confounding factors are evenly distributed between the groups given a sufficiently large sample size. The participants should be blinded to the treatment, and the investigators blinded to the treatment group and, preferably, the assessment of results.

Advantage	Disadvantage
Gold standard for evaluation of the effect of an intervention. Randomization provides the least bias in study results	Resources (time and cost)
Randomization gives the best distribution of known and unknown confounding factors between the study groups given the study has a sufficient number of participants	Recruitment of volunteers (possible selection bias)
'Blinding' is possible and best	Ethical problems – for example, difficulty in blinding in clinical studies and hiding knowledge of treatments being investigated

Table 5. Cross-sectional study

Cross-sectional study	
A group of people is identified, and data is collected in a health screening. This can be as the first step of a prospective cohort study or a study to collect information on the prevalence of risk factors or a disease.	
Advantage	**Disadvantage**
It is relatively cheap and simple to perform	It cannot reveal causal relationships
Collection of different kinds of data from participants, including anamnestic information	
It can start screening for a cohort study	
Comparison of groups of participants and analysis for associations	
Map distribution of relevant participants – for example, estimation of prevalence (how many have a specific condition in a defined period [month/year])	
Generation of hypotheses	

Systematic literature search

The number of published research papers has increased enormously; therefore, a systematic approach is of great value for researchers to identify the studies of greatest relevance to the problem being investigated. A well described systematic search for scientific literature which has been assessed in a systematic and reproducible manner is therefore important. The SRs summarizing the effect across several studies have become important in supporting decision-making in public health systems worldwide.

Systematic review

A clear description of how the literature search has been performed provides a transparent information platform of value for other researchers. Systematic reviews are also termed secondary research and is a worldwide activity through health technology assessment (HTA), Cochrane, and other international collaborations (4, 5). HTA started with technology assessment in the US in 1972 (4). Certain criteria are important in carrying out and presenting sound scientific evidence. In short, a literature search is defined and carried out in relevant databases such as PubMed, Embase, or Cinahl. It must define the population, intervention, comparator, the outcome(s), and study design; see the text on PICOS below. The result of the literature search is reviewed independently by two researchers on title level, then on abstract level, and finally the full text article(s). The effect results of the identified studies are assembled and a meta-analysis is preferably carried out. Special to HTA the results of the SR are put in context of other relevant subjects important to the health issue in question as law, ethics, economics, personnel, and/or other resources (4, 5). This method of finding the best available evidence has increased in importance and is used in this work to establish the best knowledge that can form the foundation in health policy documents for health authorities.

PICOS

Inclusion and exclusion criteria put limits on the studies included in the scientific basis of the SRs, and these criteria and other limiting factors must be reported to provide the necessary methodological transparency. Results of relevant studies are included only when they fulfil the inclusion criteria defining the population (P), intervention/risk factor (I), comparator (C), outcome (O), and study design (S). In short, these are called PICOS. This structure is of great use and importance when conducting a literature search spanning many databases.

- ❖ The **population** of each study needs to be a sufficient size. However, an advantage of the meta-analysis strategy is that small, medium, and large studies can be analysed together, giving a result based on a more diverse population than in a single study, and for this reason, the results can be more generalizable.
- ❖ **Intervention/risk factors** need to be clearly defined in each study so researchers can be confident that the studies are comparable, with the same (or very nearly the same) intervention.
- ❖ The **comparator** is important, as the effect of a measure needs to be compared to another intervention, the standard treatment, or no treatment/placebo. A comparison is needed to make valuable conclusions.
- ❖ The **outcome** varies in terms of studying oral infections and systemic diseases. Diagnostic accuracy of the included studies is important. Validated sources are public registries such as disease-specific registries, hospital data, cause-of-death registries, cancer registries, and many others. Registries of specific medical specialities based on national obligatory reporting provide valid data. In addition, the careful mapping of disease in hospitals provides coverage of relevant outcomes.
- ❖ The **study design** needs to be the same in each meta-analysis. In the hierarchy of study designs, RCTs are ranked the highest, as they have the least bias. SRs of RCTs are highly valued. Ideally, treatment studies designed as RCTs should be performed and followed prospectively to learn more about the long-term effects of the treatment.

Prospective cohorts or case-control studies with clinical or epidemiological data are good choices. Regarding a temporal relationship, the prospective follow-up of a cohort study is important, as the risk factor is measured independently of a later outcome. Case-control studies are important in studying rare diseases but may suffer from information bias and difficulty in identifying cases and controls. SRs involve these types of studies as well. In an SR, the included studies must be of the same study design, as there are inherent differences between the study designs that may influence the measured effect.

Meta-analysis and heterogeneity

Meta-analysis is a statistical method used to summarize results across several studies in SRs. The effect estimates can be relative risk (RR) or odds ratios (ORs) with 95% confidence intervals (CIs) for dichotomous outcomes. For continuous variables, the outcome standardized mean difference (SMD) or weighted mean difference (WMD) can be used. Included in the analysis is I^2 – a measure of the heterogeneity of studies. If I^2 is approximately 60% or higher, the heterogeneity is high and the studies need to be reexamined to provide an explanation. A useful supplementary analysis is the funnel plot to get an indication of publication bias of studies.

Bias

Possible causes of bias need to be explored before and during a study to minimize risks, but bias cannot always be avoided. The main causes of bias are as follows:

- ❖ Information bias due to large error margins in measurements
- ❖ Selection bias due to errors in the selection process of the study population
- ❖ Confounding due to a lack of information about factors that influence the exposure and the health outcome

Confounders

Smoking is the most well-documented risk factor, and stop-smoking campaigns are successful based on the best scientific evidence. Smoking causes cancer of the lungs, oral cavity, and urinary tract and is associated with other cancers and diseases. However, does it affect results when seemingly competing risk factors are examined? The following is a relevant example: The relation between smoking and cancer is apparent in the analyses of The Health Professionals Follow-Up Study (HPFS) (6). All risk estimates for cancer by history of periodontal disease or tooth extraction in this prospective study of 17 years follow-up were adjusted for several confounding factors including smoking. Adding smoking reduced the effect estimate for total cancer, as well as lung, oropharyngeal, stomach, pancreas, colorectal, and bladder cancers. No changes were observed for cancer of haematopoietic tissue, brain cancer, and melanoma. Periodontal infection was statistically significant when adjusting for smoking and, therefore, independent of smoking. This also applied to total cancer, as well as lung, pancreas, and kidney cancers.

Summary of available studies by study design

Table 6 presents an overview of study types forming the evidence between cause and disease as presented in the different chapters of this book.

Table 6. Overview of evidence level by different study designs for each systemic disease

Disease	Study design			
	Syste-matic review	Prospective cohort	Case control	Randomized controlled trial
Mortality	+	+		
Cardiovascular disease/myocardial infarction/ischaemic heart disease	+	+	+	+ Intermediate factors
Stroke	+	+	+	
Infective endocarditis		+	+	
Peripheral arterial disease	+	+		
Diabetes	+	+	+	+
Lung diseases	+	+	+	+
Cancer	+	+	+	
Rheumatic arthritis	+	+	+	
Pregnancy and preterm birth	+	+	+	+
Alzheimer's disease		+	+	
Gastric ulcer		+		

Concluding remarks

The different study designs have their advantages and disadvantages. Some care should be taken when interpreting the study results, as the differences observed between studies may be due to different forms of bias and/or unknown confounding factors. The inherent heterogeneity in populations and the definition of the included risk factor varies among the studies. However, the results of the numerous studies, notwithstanding their differences, may point in the same direction. More research is needed, and other studies may seek to explore the pathophysiology, microbiology, or immunology perspective.

References

1.   Matilla, KJ, Valtonen, VV, Nieminen, MS, and Asikainen, S. 1998. "Role of Infection as a Risk Factor for Atherosclerosis, Myocardial Infarction, and Stroke." *Clinical Infectious Diseases*, No. 26: 719–734.

2.   Thelle, DS. 2015. *Epidemiology: A Basis for Public Health and Disease Prevention*. Oslo: Gyldendal Akademisk.

3.   Rothman, KJ. 2002. *Epidemiology: An Introduction*. New York, NY: Oxford University Press.

4.   European Network for Health Technology Assessment. 2021. Accessed 10 September, 2021. https://eunethta.eu/

5.   Cochrane Library. https://www.cochranelibrary.com/cdsr/about-cdsr

6.   Michaud, DS, Liu, Y, Meyer, M, Giovannucci, E, and Joshipura, K. 2008 "Disease, Tooth Loss and Cancer Risk in a Prospective Study of Male Health Professionals." Lancet Oncology, No. 9: 550–558. https://dx.doi.org/10.1016/S1470-2045(08)70106-2

PART 2:

SYSTEMIC DISEASES

CHAPTER 4

ALL-CAUSE MORTALITY

Is there an association between oral infections and mortality? How is this possible? What is the modus operandi? How can there be a 'mechanism' that transfers a risk factor from one part to the rest of the body that could be in the causal chain of mortality? Is there more than one factor or even a chain of pathophysiological events? If this is the case, then can these events be prevented? What if these results are false or misinterpreted, a result due to reverse causality or simply chance? Have the right causes or associations been discovered? Are researchers using the best methods to obtain the best answer to the research question of how oral health may be a cause of mortality?

Mortality is reported as total, all cause, or cause specific in official statistics in every country. Oral health is measured in different ways, and this makes it difficult to compare studies. However, all studies are important in proving or discarding the association between oral infections and mortality as more information that may help to understand the pathologic mechanisms becomes available.

Some historic references

Oral health is very much linked to infections, how they spread, and how to limit this spread. The following are the first studies to report on oral health and total mortality. In 1823, Rayer introduced the infection hypothesis of the observed thickening with calcification of the arteries (1). He termed it 'ossification morbide.' This caused stiffening of the arteries and affected cardiovascular health. The idea was novel and did not bring much attention. Later, in 1908, Osler described atherosclerosis and causal factors, and he is considered the first to present the infection hypothesis. The four factors he described as important were 'normal wear and tear of life, the acute infections, the intoxications (including smoking, DM, [and] obesity), and the combinations of circumstances that keep blood tension high'. Osler also described fatty streaks in the atheroma. He observed a high prevalence in children, which was demonstrated in a later autopsy study (1).

Later in the twentieth century, animal studies were performed to investigate what could initiate atherosclerosis – for example, a cholesterol-rich diet. Furthermore, periopathogens were inoculated into rabbits, which caused changes on the electrocardiogram, and bacteria interacted with platelets in thrombus formation (1). More circumstantial evidence evolved during World War II. The dentist Toverud in Norway published how the dental health in school children improved with a low sugar diet during the war (1). Many other food items and cigarettes were also scarce during the war, and there was a decline in CVD that lasted even for some time after the war ended.

Official statistics are used in research to study risk factors for causes of mortality. This is common in cardiovascular and cancer research and for other diseases. Results from large cohort studies show significant trends between causes and mortality, and oral health is one of these factors. Such studies form the basis for important public health advice. In the following, results regarding oral health and its relation to mortality is given. Oral health is reported mainly by number of tooth extractions or by periodontitis in studies on mortality.

Scientific evidence

Several researchers have addressed the risk of poor health and mortality (2–12). In 2003, Tuominen, Reunanen, Paunio, Paunio et al. reported no association between oral health indicators and coronary heart disease (CHD) (2). Two years later, a large Chinese cohort study reported that tooth loss was associated with several outcomes, such as total mortality, cancer of upper gastrointestinal tract, heart disease, and stroke (3). Söder, Jin, Klinge, and Söder studied the risk of periodontitis and premature death (4). Studies geographically far apart (ranging from Scotland, Finland, Japan, Norway, Korea, Denmark, to Northern Germany) reported the same association between poor oral health and mortality (5–12). The results point in the direction of strong and less strong associations. Some studies show a "dose-response pattern" as the risk increases with an increasing number of teeth lost.

Tooth loss

Koka and Gupta conducted an SR including 49 studies in 2018 to assess the association of tooth count and mortality (13). Their aim was to study if preserving teeth influences mortality. They found a great degree of heterogeneity among the studies with regard to the definition of the tooth count variable, size of the study population, length of follow-up (from 1 to 56 years), and differences in confounders and mediators included in the analyses. Given these limitations, the authors concluded there is an association between reduced tooth count and increased risk of mortality. The limitations and heterogeneity found in the studies suggest more research of large, well-designed cohorts is needed.

In 2019, Peng, Song, Han, Chen et al. conducted an SR of 18 prospective studies involving an association between number of tooth loss and mortality from all causes, CVDs, or CHD published in the period 2003–2016 (14). Of all the studies, 15 investigated all-cause mortality (19,577 cases among 306,807 participants), while 7 (1,899 cases among 46,130 participants) explored CHD mortality and 5 (1,526 cases among 125,716 participants) focussed on CVD mortality. The included studies were conducted in Europe, Asia, North America, and Australia. Peng, Song, Han, Chen et al. found a dose-response relation between number of tooth loss and all-cause mortality of RR stratified per 10 teeth lost (RR = 1.15 [1.11–1.19]), per 20 teeth lost (RR = 1.33 [1.23–1.29]), and per 32 teeth lost (RR = 1.57 [1.39–1.51]). These results represent a significant relation for each step, although the differences between them are not large (linear trend, p = 0.306). The equivalent RR values for tooth loss for CVD were RR = 1.21 (1.01–1.44), RR = 1.45 (1.02–2.07), and RR = 1.83 (1.04–3.21) for 10, 20, and 32 teeth lost, respectively. The equivalent RR for tooth loss for CHD were RR = 1.21 (1.00–1.47), RR = 1.47 (0.99–2.17), and RR = 1.87 (1.01–3.47) for 10, 20, and 32 teeth lost, respectively. A linear trend for tooth loss was not found for CHD (p = 0.355) or CVD (p = 0.806). The meta-analyses displayed a large degree of heterogeneity (above 79%).

These results point in the same direction of a dose-response and temporal relationship between tooth loss and mortality but do not explain a direct causal relationship. Still, tooth loss is mainly caused by infections. Periodontal infection especially has a long and intermittent course through life unless treated and is further limited and prevented by optimal oral hygiene measures.

Prevention by oral hygiene measures

In the previous section, tooth loss is found to be a risk factor for mortality. Tooth loss is mainly due to infections such as gingivitis developing into periodontitis and caries developing into apical periodontitis. These conditions are, in general, preventable by standard tooth brushing, interdental cleaning, regular dental visits, fluoride usage as by fluoride tooth paste, fluoride tablets, natural or added drinking water fluoridation, fluoride rinse, or fluoride gel application. The use of dentures or implants reflects former tooth extraction. To investigate if these oral care measures are related to mortality, Hayasaka, Tomata, Aida, Watanabe et al. followed 21,730 persons aged 65 years or older, in Ōsaki City, Japan, for four years (2006–2010) (15). At the baseline survey, the authors collected data on the number of remaining teeth and on oral care measures. Data on confounding factors (such as age, gender, smoking, alcohol drinking, medical history, physical activity, psychological stress, and specific food intake) was registered. Mortality data was official information. The follow-up analyses by Cox methodology indicated the number of remaining teeth to be inversely related to mortality (p trend < 0.001). In participants with 0 to 19 teeth, oral care was inversely related to mortality. Participants practising the three types of oral care (tooth brushing, regular dental visit, and the use of dentures) had a hazard ratio (HR) of 0.54 (95% CI 0.45–0.64), compared to those who did not perform these oral care measures. A clear inverse relationship was observed for the benefit of attaining optimal oral care.

Studying participants from different populations within a country, a group of countries, or continents is useful to determine if a problem is not a local health problem and can be generalized. To compare to the Japanese study is an Iranian study by Vogtmann, Etemadi, Kamangar, Islami et al. – the Golestan Cohort Study (2004–2008) (16). A total of 50,045 persons aged 40 to 75 years took part. They were screened for tooth loss and decayed and filled teeth (commonly called decayed, missing, and filled teeth [DMFT]). Self-reported information included frequency of tooth brushing and the use of dentures. Follow-up on mortality lasted until March 2014. The authors found that the greatest tooth loss compared to those with least had an HR of 1.43 (95% CI 1.28–1.61). A similar HR was found for the DMFT score. The authors also analysed for cause-specific mortality with regard to tooth loss and found the following on mortality from CVD (HR =1.33, 95% CI 1.13–1.56), cancer (HR = 1.30, 95% CI 1.0–1.65), and injuries (HR = 1.99, 95% CI 1.28–3.09). The result for injuries was attenuated after removing persons with comorbidity at baseline.

Paganini-Hill, White, and Atchison investigated oral and general health and mortality in 5,611 elderly persons in the period 1992–2009 (median 9 years) (19). Cox regression was used to estimate the HR for men and women separately. The authors found that tooth brushing in the evening, using dental floss, and visiting the dentist were significant factors for longevity. Never brushing teeth at night increased risk by 20%–35% compared to brushing every day. Never using floss compared to using floss every day increased risk by 30%. No dental exam by a dentist within the last 12 months increased risk by 30%–50%. Lastly, edentulous persons even with dentures had a 30% higher risk of death compared to person with more than 20 teeth. The results of this study make it apparent that optimal oral health is a large health advantage measured against mortality.

Concluding remarks

All-cause mortality is the most diverse outcome in epidemiologic research. As it includes all causes predicting diseases, it is affected by the availability of health resources of all kinds through an individual's lifespan; living conditions, including the availability of a sound diet and smoking; and many factors influencing the socioeconomic status of individuals in any country. Therefore, it is important to have well-conducted studies worldwide identifying the risk posed by poor oral health, tooth extractions, and chronic periodontitis over and above known risk factors to realise this is a world health problem.

References

1.   Håheim, Lise L. 2014. "The Infection Hypothesis Revisited: Oral Infections and Cardiovascular Diseases." *Epidemiology Research International*, No. 2014: 735378. https://doi.org/10.1155/2014/735378
2.   Tuominen, R, Reunanen, A, Paunio, M, Paunio, I, and Aromaa, A. 2003. "Oral Health Indicators Poorly Predict Coronary Heart Disease Deaths." *Journal of Dental Research*, No. 82: 713–718.
3.   Abnet, CC, Qiao, YL, Dawsey, SM, Dong, Z-W, Taylor, PR, and Mark, SD. 2005. Tooth Loss Is Associated with Increased Risk of Total Death and Death from Upper Gastrointestinal Cancer, Heart Disease, and Stroke in a Chinese Population-Based Cohort." *International Journal of Epidemiology*, No. 34: 467–474.
4.   Söder, B, Jin, LJ, Klinge, B, and Söder, PO. 2007. "Periodontitis and Premature Death: A 16-Year Longitudinal Study in a Swedish Urban Population." *Journal of Periodontal Research*, No. 42: 361–366.
5.   Tu, YK, Galobardes, B, Smith, GD, McCarron, P, Jeffreys, M, and Gilthorp, MS. 2007. "Associations between Tooth Loss and Mortality Patterns in the Glasgow Alumni Cohort." *Heart*, No. 93: 1098–1103.

6. Heitmann, BL, and Gamborg, M. 2008. "Remaining Teeth, Cardiovascular Morbidity and Death among Adult Danes." *Preventive Medicine*, No. 47: 156–160.

7. Choe, H, Kim, YH, Park, JW, Kim, SY, Lee, S-L, and Jee, SH. 2009. "Tooth Loss, Hypertension and Risk for Stroke in a Korean Population." *Atherosclerosis*, No. 203: 550–556.

8. Watt, RG, Tsakos, G, de Oliveira, C, and Hamer, M. 2012. "Tooth Loss and Cardiovascular Disease Mortality Risk – Results from the Scottish Health Survey." *PLoS One*, No. 7: e30797.

9. Schwahn, C, Polzer, I, Haring, R, Dörr, M, Wallaschofski, H, Kocher, T, Mundt, T, Holtfreter, B, Samietz, S, Völzke, H, and Biffar R. 2013. "Missing, Unreplaced Teeth and Risk of All-Cause and Cardiovascular Mortality." *International Journal of Cardiology*, No. 167 (4): 1430–1437.
https://doi.org/10.1016/ j.ijcard.2012.04.061

10. Hirotomi, T, Yoshihara, A, Ogawa, H, and Miyazaki, H. 2015. "Number of Teeth and 5-Year Mortality in an Elderly Population." *Community Dentistry and Oral Epidemiology*, No. 43: 226–231.

11. Liljestrand, JM, Havulinna, AS, Paju, S, Männistö, S, Salomaa, V, and Pussinen, PJ. 2015. "Missing Teeth Predict Incident Cardiovascular Events, Diabetes, and Death." *Journal of Dental Research*, No. 94: 1055–1062.

12. Håheim, Lise L, Rønningen, KS, Nafstad, P, Schwarze, PE, Thelle, DS, and Olsen, I. 2017. "Number of Tooth Extractions Is Associated with Increased Risk of Mortality." *SciTz Dentistry: Research & Therapy*, No. 2 (1).

13. Koka, S, and Gupta, A. 2018. "Association between Missing Tooth Count and Mortality: A Systematic Review." *Journal of Prosthodontic Research*, No. 62 (2): 134–151.
https://doi.org/10.1016/j.jpor.2017.08.003

14. Peng, J, Song, J, Han, J, Chen, Z, Yin, X, Zhu, J, and Song, J. 2019. "The Relationship between Tooth Loss and Mortality from All Causes, Cardiovascular Diseases, and Coronary Heart Disease in the General Population: Systematic Review and Dose-Response Meta-analysis of Prospective Cohort Studies." *Bioscience Reports*, No. 39 (1): BSR20181773. https://doi.org/10.1042/BSR20181773

15. Hayasaka, K, Tomata, Y, Aida, J, Watanabe, T, Kakizaki, M, and Tsuji, I. 2013. "Tooth Loss and Mortality in Elderly Japanese Adults: Effect of Oral Care." *Journal of the American Geriatrics Society*, No. 61 (5): 815–820. https://doi.org/10.1111/jgs.12225

16. Vogtmann, E, Etemadi, A, Kamangar, F, Islami, F, Roshandel, G, Poustchi, H, Pourshams, A, Khoshnia, M, Gharravi, A, Brennan, PJ, Boffetta, P, Dawsey, SM, Malekzadeh, R, and Abnet, CC. 2017. "Oral Health and Mortality in the Golestan Cohort Study." *International Journal of Epidemiology*, No. 46 (6): 2028–2035. https://doi.org/10.1093/ije/dyx056

17. Farquhar, DR, Divaris, K, Mazul, AL, Weissler, MC, Zevallos, JP, and Olshan, AF. 2017. "Poor Oral Health Affects Survival in Head and Neck Cancer." *Oral Oncology*, No. 73: 111–117. https://doi.org/10.1016/j.oraloncology.2017.08.009

18. Chang, CC, Lee, WT, Hsiao, JR, Ou, CY, Huang, CC, Tsai, ST, Chen, KC, Huang, JS, Wong, TY, Lai, YH, Wu, YH, Hsueh, WT, Wu, SY, Yen, CJ, Chang, JY, Lin, CL, Weng, YL, Yang, HC, Chen, YS, and Chang, JS. 2019. "Oral Hygiene and the Overall Survival of Head and Neck Cancer Patients." *Cancer Medicine*, No. 8 (4): 1854–1864. https://doi.org/10.1002/cam4.2059

19. Paganini-Hill, A, White, SC, and Atchison, KA. 2011. "Dental Health Behaviours, Dentition, and Mortality in the Elderly: The Leisure World Cohort Study." *Journal of Aging Research*, No. 2011: 156061. https://doi.org/10.4061/2011/156061

CHAPTER 5

CARDIOVASCULAR DISEASES/MYOCARDIAL INFARCTION/ISCHAEMIC HEART DISEASE

CVDs constitute a range of conditions, and they are dominant causes of disease and mortality worldwide (https://www.who.int/news-room/fact-sheets/detail/the-top-10-causes-of-death). CVD is considered to be a noncommunicable disorder and to be multicausal, as shown in numerous studies on cause, effect of treatment and prevention, follow-up studies, and reports from national registry data. Oral infections are not included in the list of causes for CVD by the WHO, but there is ample scientific evidence for a change, as reported by the Joint European Federation of Periodontology (EFP)/AAP Workshop on Periodontitis and atherosclerotic CVD in 2013 (1). In December 2020, the World Health Assembly (WHA) suggested including health as part of WHO's noncommunicable diseases and universal health coverage agendas. The WHA included oral health as one of the noncommunicable diseases in May 2021. (https://www.who.int/news/item/27-05-2021-world-health-assembly-resolution-paves-the-way-for-better-oral-health-care)

It has been, and still is, of great importance to study the causes of CVD and the effect of prophylactic measures and treatment. Primary prevention includes measures for healthy living shown to reduce the risk, such as smoking cessation, regular physical exercise, a diet with low levels of animal fat and sugar, more vegetables, and modest alcohol consumption. Main pharmacological treatments include blood pressure–lowering drugs, cholesterol-lowering drugs (e.g. statins), and antithrombotic drugs. Treatment involves surgery, including inserting stents in the coronary arteries, performing vascular surgery, changing heart valves, or inserting pacemakers. Other important factors include a family history of CVD that may indicate hypercholesterolemia.

CVD causality is a much-studied subject, as it is a widely recurring global disease with a high mortality. Fortunately, the mortality is decreasing where modern prevention and treatment options are available. The notion of infections being partly or fully to blame was raised many years ago, and oral infections such as periodontitis, apical periodontitis, and periimplantitis have been focused on. Tooth extraction has been used as an indicator of long-standing oral infection. Oral infections are in close proximity to the circulation, and the oral cavity harbours several anaerobic bacteria. Facultative bacteria also drive infections.

The epidemiology of CVDs is far more dynamic than that of many other noncommunicable diseases with considerable social differences and rapidly changing disease risk. This pattern, which is seen worldwide, suggests that external and environmental factors play a major role in influencing the disease risk of CVDs. Low-grade inflammation is considered the most important part of atherosclerotic pathogenesis, but this concept does not explain the dynamic of the disorders. Low-grade inflammation is associated to several well-recognized cardiovascular risk factors, even if the biological link may seem obscure. What triggers low-grade inflammation? The chapters on CVDs, including MI, are attempts to link oral health to the pathogenesis of atherosclerosis. Oral health varies both within and between populations and over time. It might, therefore, be a potential explanatory variable when discussing disease variation. One of the pitfalls in medical science is the compartmentalization of the human body, and the distinction between dental medicine and that of the rest of the body has probably led to unnecessary knowledge gaps. The chapters in this book represent up-to-date knowledge and the current understanding of the atherosclerotic process, with its detrimental complications, and connects this with inflammatory processes in the oral cavity. Still, one might ask what else should be involved in the first line of defence against external factors than the oral cavity if low-grade inflammation is to be avoided. The area is open for further research, even if interventional studies with hard endpoints may seem infeasible or even unethical, but well-controlled longitudinal studies should be encouraged. There is a large number of studies seeking to firmly establish an association and possibly causality between PD and MI/CHD. In recent years, several SRs have been conducted. This chapter presents much of the evidence by SRs.

Oral infections and causal mechanisms for cardiovascular disease

How can oral bacteria be part of a causal mechanism for CVD? Buhlin explored this hypothesis in his doctoral thesis, where data from questionnaires and blood samples were used to study a wide range of characteristics of the participants (2). One analysis specifically concerned CVD in women as CVD is not common in young and middle-aged women. The analyses of the validity of self-report and self-assessment of oral health was found to be adequate and important.

Two main possible pathologic mechanisms – atherosclerosis and thrombosis – are described below. Atherosclerosis is considered to be an inflammatory disease of the arterial wall (3). Oral anaerobic bacteria and bacterial products such as LPSs have access to the circulation, which transports the bacteria and bacterial products to distant sites. The bacteria can dislodge and enter arterial walls, and bacterial DNA have been found in specimens of heart valves, arterial walls, and aortic aneurysms. Moreover, viable bacteria have been found in arterial walls. Bacterial DNA of different sources, such as the oral cavity, the gut, the environment, and the skin, have been identified in serum. The question arises as to why the immune system does not manage to stop this bacterial intrusion from the oral cavity and other infections. Studies have analysed and found antibodies to oral bacteria in the serum, which indicates oral infections have occurred. Antibodies to bacteria and viruses are the body's main defence against infections. Antibody production varies in individuals, and some produce little amounts. These people are at increased risk – as shown in the Oslo II Study, where a low level of the oral anaerobe bacterium *Tannerella forsythia* predicted CVD mortality in men with a history of MI (4).

Atherosclerosis

Atherosclerosis is a disease of the arteries. It is an inflammatory condition that gradually develops with deposits in the wall and lumen of the arteries at different stages. Tuomainen's 2009 doctoral thesis provides an overview of the pathology of atherosclerosis induced by bacteria (3). The author offers a complex pathway with several mechanisms, and possibly more have been revealed in more recent research.

The arterial wall consists of three layers (Figure 1): The first is the inner layer – intima. It is next to the lumen and is a layer of endothelial cells with an internal elastic lamina. It consists mainly of extracellular matrix components, collagen, and proteoglycans. The middle layer – media – contains smooth muscle cells. The third layer – adventitia – is composed of connective tissues, as well as fibroblasts and smooth muscle cells.

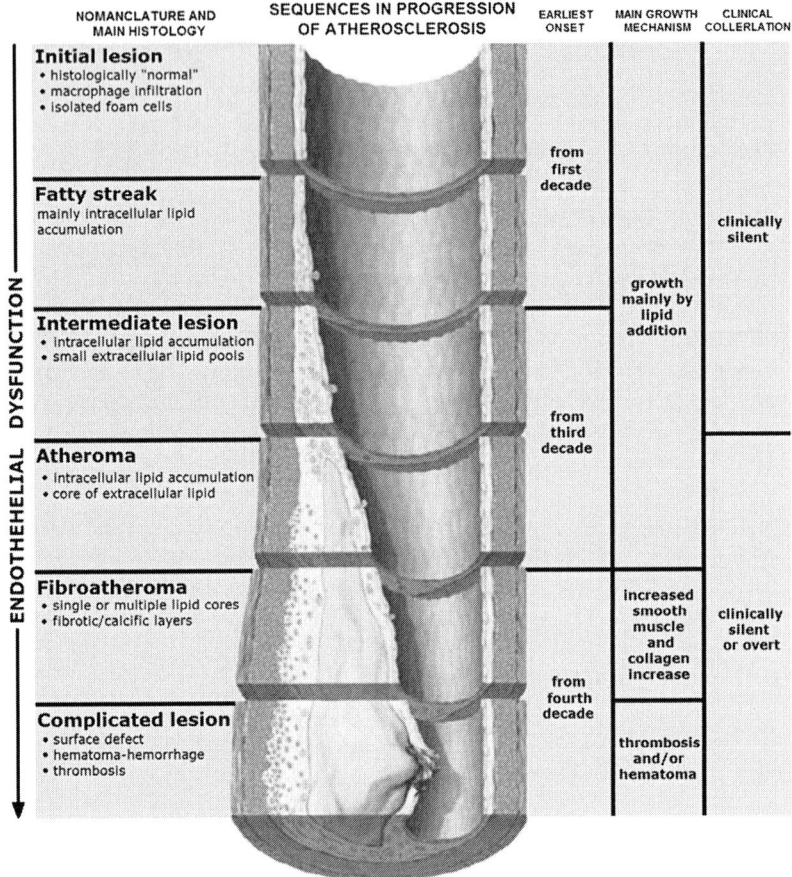

Figure 1. Schematic presentation of the development of atherosclerosis if uninterrupted. The figure presents the common nomenclature and is an illustrative presentation to identify the different pathological stages of atherosclerosis. Source: https://en.wikipedia.org/wiki/Atherosclerosis

The initial formation of atherosclerosis can be divided into five stages:

- ❖ The first stage involves the adhesion of monocytes to the arterial wall. Normally, vessels can resist this adhesion, but monocytes may adhere due to lipid accumulation, smoking, microbes, insulin resistance, hypertension, proinflammatory cytokines such as TNF-α and IL-1 beta, and endothelial cells expressing adhesion molecules.

❖ After the endothelial binding, monocytes are recruited into the intima media of the arterial wall and accumulate.
❖ Monocytes mature to macrophages and proliferate.
❖ Macrophages accumulate cholesterol ester and develop into cells termed foam cells.
❖ The foam cells transform into fatty streaks. The development may stop here or progress to advanced lesions of atherosclerosis.

Atherosclerosis progress with the accumulation of lipid and immune cells in the intima layer forming "fatty streaks" (Figure 1). These can be identified in young and old people, indicating an early start in life for atherosclerosis in susceptible individuals. In fatty streaks, foam cells which are lipid-laden macrophages develop. The fatty streaks may develop further to atheroma with more foam cells, fibroblasts, and lipid droplets. As atheroma develops, a fibrous cap forms towards the lumen, which consists of fibroblasts and smooth muscle cells. The lesion grows towards adventitia and towards the arterial lumen. Monocytes can enter the atheroma, and cell proliferation causes increasing sizes of the atherosclerotic lesions. The atheroma can grow until it causes the obstruction of the artery. These lesions can also rupture and release their content into the bloodstream. The circulating elements contribute to thrombus formation, clot formation, and emboli being lodged in distant arteries, causing infarcts.

Central to the understanding of the development of atherosclerosis is the knowledge of lipid transport and metabolism. Different lipoproteins, consisting of lipids and apolipoproteins, transport cholesterol. There are five different categories: chylomicrons, very low density lipoproteins, intermediate density lipoproteins, low density lipoproteins (LDLs), and high density lipoproteins (HDLs). Cholesterol comes with diet, exogenously, and is also synthesized, endogenously. About two thirds of available cholesterol is carried by LDLs and is the source of steroidogenesis and cellular membranes. The liver clears LDLs, but if the level is high, LDLs remain in the circulation. Some cell types, such as macrophages, can take up cholesterol, causing an accumulation in arterial walls. An additional mechanism is the transport of cholesterol by HDLs from peripheral tissues to the liver. This process is called reverse cholesterol transport.

Atherosclerosis in arterial vessel walls is a persistent inflammation. In the atheroma, further biological processes, including calcification, may occur, and the fibrous cap may rupture and become an emboli, as mentioned earlier (2).

As fibrous material deposits and calcification occur, the lumen of the arteries gradually gets narrower as the arterial wall thickens, and the atheroma stage develops. A thrombus can form, and at some point, the lesion may burst. This can have serious consequences in the form of resultant emboli being transported by the bloodstream and deposited in smaller arteries, causing infarcts at distant sites. Occlusion of these arteries can occur due to the gradual build-up of atherosclerosis in the vessel wall and the added thrombosis from a distant site. The coronary arteries are prone to atherosclerosis, causing MI. In addition, major sites such as the descending aorta is prone to developing aneurysm and the bifurcation of the external carotid artery is a site prone to obstruction and emboli causing stroke.

Thrombosis

Thrombus formation is dependent on platelets and protein clotting factors. When blood vessels are damaged, the body immediately responds by constricting vessels, fibrin is formed at the injured site to stop bleeding, and platelets accumulate at the injured site to aid the healing of the injury. Thrombosis consists of platelets that adhere to each other, and later, fibrous materials hold them together.

Thrombosis mainly occurs in veins but also occurs in arteries. If the leg muscles do not pump blood through the veins, thrombi may slowly form in the deep veins of the legs. The blood flow changes, and platelets accumulate. The platelets form thrombi, which may release smaller parts as emboli that may get lodged in the lungs. Damaged heart valves, septal foramen, or other heart deformations can be sites for thrombus formation and become the source of emboli that dislodge and may cause cerebral infarction. Bacteria are known to influence this process and have been shown to influence the adherence of platelets in the formation of thrombi (5).

Immunity

Immunity is involved by both innate and adaptive processes in atherosclerosis. The innate immune response is nonspecific and identifies pathogen-associated molecular patterns such as LPSs and modified LDLs. Macrophages have toll-like receptors and scavenger receptors and release cytokines and adhesion molecules, which affect the inflammatory status of arterial walls. The adaptive immunity system is slower, as it involves T- and B-cells, and requires antigen-presenting cells (such as dendritic cells and macrophages) that present antigens to T-cells, which then initiate a response to the antigens. The cytotoxic T-cells can then attack any cell with presenting antigens. The T-cell reaction is an early immunological response but not necessarily an early stage in atherosclerosis.

Results from epidemiologic studies on cardiovascular disease risk

Single studies (cross-sectional or prospective)

Beck, Garcia, Heiss, Vokonas et al. wanted to study if there was an association between an underlying immune trait in persons with chronic PD and the development of atherosclerosis (10). In addition to the infection, the body produces several inflammatory and immunological substances as endotoxin (LPS) and inflammatory cytokines (especially Thromboxane A2 (TXA2), IL-1β, prostaglandin E2, and TNF-α), which serve to initiate and exacerbate atherogenesis and thromboembolic events. The authors used the combined data from the Normative Aging Study and the Dental Longitudinal Study, sponsored by the U.S. Department of Veterans Affairs. Periodontal measurements were mean bone loss scores, and worst probing pocket depth scores per tooth were measured in 1,147 men between 1968 and 1971. During the follow-up, 207 men developed CHD, 59 died of CHD, and 40 had strokes. Adjusted for CVD risk factors, the ORs were 1.5, 1.9, and 2.8 for bone loss and total CHD, fatal CHD, and stroke, respectively.

The Oral Infections and Vascular Disease Epidemiology Study was a study on the association between periodontal status and CVD with a broad approach (15–17). In the first publication, the researchers presented results on the relationship between PD, tooth loss, and carotid artery plaque. They enrolled 711 persons (mean age 66 +/- 9 years) with no history of stroke or MI. As expected, periodontitis was more severe with increasing tooth loss. Prevalence of carotid artery plaque was 60% among those with ≥ 10 missing teeth versus 46% for those with 0–9 missing teeth. In the second publication of the Oral Infections and Vascular Disease Epidemiology Study, periodontal pathogens and hypertension is reported for 653 dentate men and women. Hypertension was considered as systolic blood pressure (SBP) ≥ 140 mmHg and diastolic blood pressure (DBP) ≥ 90 mmHg, or taking antihypertensive medication, or through self-reported history. The researchers found that the etiologic bacterial burden was positively associated with both blood pressure and prevalent hypertension. The third publication that reported on the relationship of periodontal bacteria and subclinical atherosclerosis involved a cross-sectional study design (15–17). In all, 1,056 persons (mean age 69 years +/- 9 years) were included. The examination included bacterial analyses of subgingival plaque by DNA-DNA checkerboard hybridization of 11 known periodontal bacteria. Subclinical atherosclerosis was estimated by a carotid scan with high-resolution B-mode ultrasound to estimate intima-media thickness (IMT). White blood cell count and C-reactive protein (CRP) values, as well as other known risk factors for CVD, were obtained. An analysis of mean carotid artery IMT across three levels of periodontal bacterial burden was modelled. The significant association of overall bacterial burden with IMT was independent of CRP. The authors concluded from the results that their study provides evidence of a direct relationship between periodontal microbiology and subclinical atherosclerosis.

Yu, Chasman, Buring, Rose et al. conducted a large prospective cohort study (18). They studied if incident periodontitis influences future risk of vascular diseases. The researchers compared cardiovascular risk of prevalent PD with new incident cases. The outcomes were major CVDs, MI, ischaemic stroke, and total CVD. A total of 39,863 predominantly white women (age $\geq$ 45 years) who did not report CVD at the screening were included in the study. The cohort was followed for 15.7 years on average. Prevalent cases were 18%, incident cases were 7.3%, and never cases were 74.7%. Incidence rates of all CVD outcomes were higher in women with prevalent or incident PD. For women with incident PD, risk factor–adjusted HRs were 1.42 (95% CI 1.14–1.77) for major CVD, 1.72 (1.25–2.38) for MI, 1.41 (1.02–1.95) for ischaemic stroke, and 1.27 (1.06–1.52) for total CVD compared to never PD. The same was observed for women with prevalent PD: adjusted HRs were 1.14 (1.00–1.31) for major CVD, 1.27 (1.04–1.56) for MI, 1.12 (0.91–1.37) for ischaemic stroke, and 1.15 (1.03–1.28) for total CVD.

A Finnish study investigated the prediction of serum matrix metalloproteinase (MMP) 8 concentration in 1,018 men with no CVD in a 10-year follow-up (19). MMP-8 is involved in not only the breakdown of extracellular matrix during tissue repair but also pathogenic situations of RA, periodontitis, and atherosclerosis. It is also involved in immune response. Elevated MMP-8 in men with no CVD at baseline had elevated risk for fatal CVD outcomes as CHD, CVD, and all-cause mortality.

The Scottish Health Survey was a population-based survey that included 11,869 men and women (mean age 50 years) (20, 21). The survey data were linked to clinical hospital records for CVD events and death over an eight-year follow-up. The researchers examined whether tooth brushing was associated with CVDs. Measurements of fibrinogen (a coagulation marker) and CRP (an inflammation marker) were included. The researchers found a risk for a CVD event in a fully adjusted model (HR = 1.7, 95% CI 1.3–2.3, p < 0.001).

The National FINRISK Study (1997) included 8,446 persons in a population-based study with a 13-year follow-up (22). Screening data included missing teeth as part of a dental status, and data on all-cause death, CVD events, and diabetes was obtained from official registries. In the follow-up analyses, the researchers found that having ≥ five teeth missing was associated with 60% to 140% increased hazard for incident CHD events (P < 0.020) and acute MI (P < 0.010). Incident CVD (P < 0.043), diabetes (P < 0.040), and death of any cause (P < 0.019) were associated with ≥ nine missing teeth. No association with stroke was observed."

In the Women's Health Initiative Observational Study (US), LaMonte, Genco, Hovey, Wallace et al. investigated the association of periodontitis and edentulism with risk of CVD events in 57,001 postmenopausal women aged 55 to 89 years (23). They were enrolled during the years 1993–1998 and asked about their oral health. The mean follow-up for CVD events was 6.7 years. During follow-up 3,589 CVD events occurred, and 3,816 women died. Periodontitis was not associated with CVD events but with total mortality (HR = 1.12, 95% CI 1.05–1.21). Edentulism was associated with risk of CVD and mortality in age- and smoking-adjusted analyses. With further adjustments for covariates, the CVD association was no longer significant, but was for mortality, HR was 1.17 (95% CI 1.02–1.33).

Several inflammatory factors are activated by inflammation and infections. Hs-CRP is considered a nonspecific inflammation indicator, indicating that it is elevated not only during infections but also in other disorders. This was explored by Håheim, Nafstad, Olsen, Schwarze et al. In their study, hs-CRP levels were compared in a range of self-reported chronic health disorders: osteoporosis, asthma, diabetes, chronic bronchitis/emphysema, MI, current oral infections, stroke, angina pectoris, hay fever, and fibromyalgia/chronic pain syndrome (24). The researchers found that men with osteoporosis presented the highest mean values (6.53 mg/l) then asthma presented an increased mean hs-CRP level of 5.01 mg/l, chronic bronchitis/emphysema 4.42 mg/l, diabetes 4.53 mg/l, men with MI 4.27 mg/l, fibromyalgia/chronic pain syndrome 4.79 mg/l. Non-cases varied between 3.53 and 3.60 mmol/l.

Systematic reviews

In 2002, Genco, Offenbacher, and Beck published a review of the epidemiology of PD and CVD, exploring the literature up to date (6). The authors included nine prospective cohort studies and found that six did show an association (Table 1) and three did not (Table 2). The studies were performed in the US, Finland, and Canada, with follow-up ranging from 6 to 23 years. Not all the studies used the same measures of PD status and development, which is a problem recognized by the researchers.

Table 1. Genco, Offenbacher, and Beck included the following studies and their statistically significant main results

First author, year (reference)	Country, years of follow-up	Periodontal disease measure	Outcome	Risk, adjusted
De Stefano, 1993 (7)	US, 15 years	Russell's periodontal index	Death from CVD	RR = 1.7
Mattila, 1995 (8)	Finland, 7 years	Total dental index	New MI or death from CHD	RR = 1.2
Joshipura, 1996 (9)	US, 6 years	Reported tooth loss due to periodontitis	Fatal MI, nonfatal MI, sudden death	RR = 1.7
Beck, 1996 (10)	US, 12 years	Whole mouth bone level	New CHD Fatal CHD Stroke	OR = 1.5 OR = 1.9 OR = 2.8
Morrison, 1999 (11)	Canada, 23 years	Mild gingivitis Severe gingivitis Periodontitis	Fatal CHD and fatal stroke	RR = 3.6 RR = 6.9 RR = 3.4
Wu, 2000 (12)	US, 21 years	Gingivitis and periodontitis (≥ 4 mm pockets) edentulous	Incidental nonhae-morrhagic stroke	RR = 1.2 gingivitis RR = 2.1 periodontitis

Table 2. Genco, Offenbacher, and Beck included the following studies and their statistically nonsignificant main results

First author, year (reference)	Country, years of follow-up	Periodontal disease measure	Outcome	Risk, adjusted
Joshipura, 1996 (9)	US, 6 years	Reported history of periodontitis	Fatal MI, nonfatal MI, sudden death	RR = 1.04
Hujoel, 2000 (13)	US, 21 years	Gingivitis and periodontitis (≥ 1 mm pockets) by Russell's periodontal index	Death or hospitalization due to CHD	HR = ns* gingivitis RR = 1.14 periodontitis
Howell, 2001 (14)	US, 12.3 years	Reported history of periodontal disease	Death from CHD, nonfatal MI, or stroke	RR = 1.01

*ns=nonsignificant

Genco, Offenbacher, and Beck also reported on evidence of case-control studies that showed periodontitis to be associated with MI and pathologic studies that showed oral bacteria present in atheroma and that some oral bacteria are associated with platelet aggregation important in thrombus formation (6).

Almeida, Fagundes, Maia, Lima et al. conducted an SR of studies focussing on Gram-negative bacteria in the oral cavity and the association with atherosclerosis in adults (25). The studies compared groups with or without periodontitis. In all, 2,138 studies were identified, and 4 cohort studies were included. The authors concluded that an association between the two disorders was observed with elevated levels of inflammatory markers, mainly CRP and IL-6. An important finding is the identification of bacteria in arterial tissue, proving the ability of bacteria to spread via the circulation, attach to the arterial wall, and penetrate the arterial walls (as in an aneurysm) and heart valves. Examples of such pathologic studies have shown oral and other bacteria can be found in stenosed cardiac valves and aneurysm of descending aorta (26, 27).

In 2002, Müller published an SR on studies exploring if chronic periodontitis played a role in the pathology of CVD and cerebrovascular diseases (28). In the abstract, the author reported on the meta-analyses of prospective studies that showed RR values of periodontitis for CHD and ischaemic stroke to be 1.12 (95% CI 0.95–1.33) and 1.73 (95% CI 0.89–3.34), respectively. These results did not indicate any positive associations between chronic periodontitis and CVD disease.

Later SRs contradicted these early results. In 2009, results from an SR of cohort, case-control, and cross-sectional studies was published, including 47 studies of 215 identified studies (29). From these epidemiological studies, Blaizot, Vergnes, Nuwwareh, Amar et al. investigated PD and CVD events; 47 studies were observational, of which 29 studies were included in the analyses. Seven studies were prospective cohorts, and 22 were case-control and cross-sectional studies. The risk estimate of the prospective studies comparing participants with PD versus those without PD was a pooled RR of 1.34, (95% CI 1.27–1.42, p < 0.0001). The combined estimate for the 22 case-control and cross-sectional studies was 2.35 (95% CI 1.87–2.96, p < 0.0001). The risk estimates of the case-control and cross-sectional studies being higher than those of the prospective studies can be due to these study designs having a higher risk of information bias in both exposure and outcome registration.

A recent review by Larvin, Kang, Aggarwal, Pavitt et al. in 2021 concerned studies of incident CVD in people with PD compared to periodontal healthy ones (30). The authors searched for prospective cohorts and RCTs for their meta-analyses. CVD outcomes included any CVD, MI, CHD, and stroke. PD status was either self-reported or clinically recorded. Diagnostic methods and severity of PD were measured either clinically or by self-report. The authors identified 32 studies, and 30 studies were included in the meta-analyses. The results were as follows:

- The risk of CVD was significantly higher in PD compared to non-PD (RR = 1.20, 95% CI 1.14–1.26).
- CVD risk did not differ between clinical and self-reported PD diagnosis (RR = 0.97, 95% CI 0.87–1.07).
- CVD risk was higher in men (RR= 1.16, 95% CI 1.08–1.25) and in severe PD cases (RR = 1.25, 95% CI 1.15–1.35).

- The risk of stroke was highest of all types of CVD (RR = 1.24, 95% CI 1.12–1.38).
- CHD risk was also increased among all types of CVD (RR = 1.14, 95% CI 1.08–1.21).

The results show consistent results of increased CVD risk by periodontal disease, whether recorded by clinical analyses or self-reported. Regarding the result on the risk of stroke being high in men, this is an indication of who will benefit the most from treatment and follow-up of periodontal treatment.

Joshi, Bapat, Anderson, Dawson et al. explored studies on the reported prevalence of periodontal microorganisms in coronary atheroma and reported on clot samples collected from patients with MI and PD (31). The researchers identified 14 eligible studies from the period 2007–2017, of which 12 reported on DNA of periodontal bacteria present in coronary athcrosclerotic plaque specimens. The most frequent periodontal microbes were *Porphyromonas gingivalis* (Pg) and *Aggregatibacter actinomycetemcomitans* (Aa), with Pg significantly more than Aa. Other microbes identified include *Pseudomonas fluorescens*, *Streptococcus* spp., and *Chlamydia pneumoniae*. The presence of oral bacterial DNA in arterial wall specimens is a clear indication of a link between oral infections and CVD. This knowledge is important in studying causality of CVD by oral infections. This confirmative evidence indicates that oral bacteria metastasize to distant organs.

Apical periodontitis is the result of caries advancing into the pulp of a tooth and spreading through the apical foramen and into the surrounding alveolar bone/the jaw. Berlin-Broner, Febbraio, and Levin explored observational studies published until 2015 on apical periodontitis and CVD risk (32). The systematic literature search identified 19 eligible studies with different study designs: 10 case-control studies, 5 cross-sectional studies, and 4 cohort studies. The quality of the study designs varied with regard to assessing causality, and prospective cohorts are considered to be the best to study the risk of future events. RCTs are best in terms of studying the effect of a treatment but are rarely followed up prospectively for a long time. The researchers report this heterogenic variation in evidence. Thirteen of the studies reported a positive association. However, five did not, and one was negative.

Periodontal disease intervention

Studies have been performed to estimate the effect of interventions by treatment of PD on CVD parameters. Those mentioned here do not represent all intervention studies. From a causal perspective, such studies, in addition to prospective cohorts especially, are important.

In 2004, D'Aiuto, Ready, and Tonetti published their study involving 94 systemically healthy persons who suffered from severe generalized periodontitis (33). At baseline, it was observed that those with the most severe periodontitis had a higher CVD risk of elevated CRP (OR = 5.6 [1.2–27.4]). After treatment, the follow-up revealed a significant decrease in CRP risk.

Since then, more studies have been published. A SR by Sharma, Sridhar, McIntosh, Messow et al. in 2021 presents results of PD treatment by intensive periodontal treatment (IPT), which included supra- and subgingival instrumentation (34). The researchers explored eight studies comparing the effects of IPT or conventional periodontal treatment on arterial blood pressure, endothelial function, and inflammatory/metabolic biomarkers (such as CRP, IL-6, IL-10, IFN-γ) and metabolic biomarkers (HDL, LDL, and triglycerides (TGs)). The results of the meta-analysis for the overall IPT effect estimates (pooled WMD) on the primary outcome for SBP and DBP was -4.3 mmHg (95% CI -9.10–0.48, p = 0.08) and -3.16 mmHg (95% CI -6.51–0.19, p = 0.06), respectively. Subgroup analyses of normotensive persons were nonsignificant. Analyses of prehypertensive/hypertensive participants strengthened the association; SBP reduction was -11.41 mmHg (95% CI -13.66–9.15). The DBP reduction was -8.43 mmHg (95% CI -10.96 to -5.91). Improvements were observed for significant modest reduction in CRP and improvement of endothelial function following IPT at all analysed timepoints. No significant change was found for IL-6, IL-10, IFN-γ, HDL, LDL, or TGs. The authors suggest in their conclusion that periodontal treatment should be accepted as part of hypertension treatment. Lowered blood pressure reduces CVD risk.

International Classification of Diseases

The International List of Causes of Death specifies different disorders and was adopted by the International Statistical Institute in 1893. Since then, several revisions of the International Classification of Diseases (ICD) framework have been published, and current version in use is the 10th revision. In 1948, the WHO was entrusted with the registry. From the sixth revision in 1948, morbidity was included. From 2022, the 11th revision will be used. The codes are used when diagnosing information of cases in hospital journals, different specific disease registries, and mortality registers (https://www.who.int/standards/classifications/classification-of-diseases). The framework serves to assure quality of the data used in general population statistics and research. ICD-10 has been cited by 20,000 researchers, and it is accepted and used in more than 150 countries. It has been translated to more than 40 languages for ease of use and serves to obtain reliable statistics worldwide that are suitable for important comparisons and ranking for important policy knowledge and decision-making.

SCORE chart and risk of cardiovascular disease issued by the European Society of Cardiology

To assist clinicians and health authorities, risk scores have been established. The Systematic Coronary Risk Evaluation (SCORE) chart, the European High Risk Chart has been developed by the European Society of Cardiology (ESC) (Figure 2) (35). (https://www.escardio.org/static-file/Escardio/About %20the%20ESC/Annual-Reports/ESCAnnualReport2020-BD.pdf)

The chart gives the 10-year risk for fatal CVD in populations in Europe based on 12 European cohort studies, 250,000 patient data sets, three million person years of observation, and 7,000 fatal cardiovascular events. SCORE separately combines these data into a high-risk score and a low-risk score, depending on the risk pattern of European countries for men and women. The factors involved are age, blood pressure, cholesterol level, and smoking. Oral infections are not included, as there are few epidemiologic studies that combine oral infections and CVD.

The ESC wrote in their 2020 report that CVD costs are enormous, amounting to an estimated €210 billion annually in the EU. A staggering 19.9 million new cases of CVD occur in the 54 ESC member countries. Prevention and treatment of heart disease is important and will be so for many years to come.

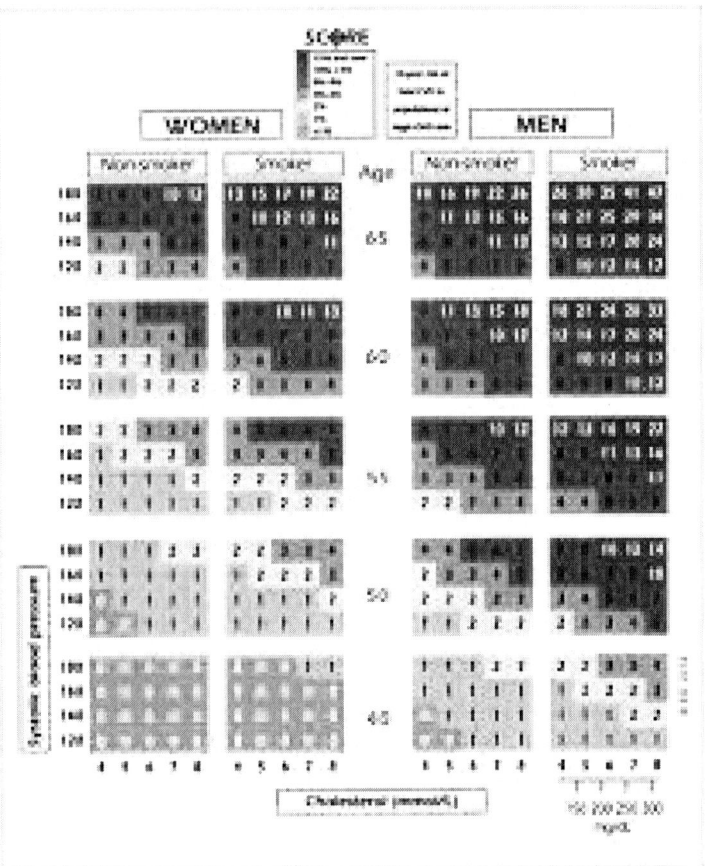

Figure 2. SCORE chart: 10-year risk of fatal cardiovascular disease in populations of countries at high cardiovascular risk based on the following risk factors: age, sex, smoking, systolic blood pressure, total cholesterol. SCORE = Systematic Coronary Risk Estimation.
Source:
https://www.google.com/search?q=score+chart+cardiovascular+risk&sxsrf=AOae mvKCoo0Mm15svhMuRBJ_KO4nw7SopA:1631694567988&tbm=isch&source

The WHO and cardiovascular disease

The WHO focuses its efforts on prevention strategies against cardiovascular disease to protect people from tobacco smoking, maintain a healthy diet, be physically active, and avoid harmful use of alcohol (Figure 3).

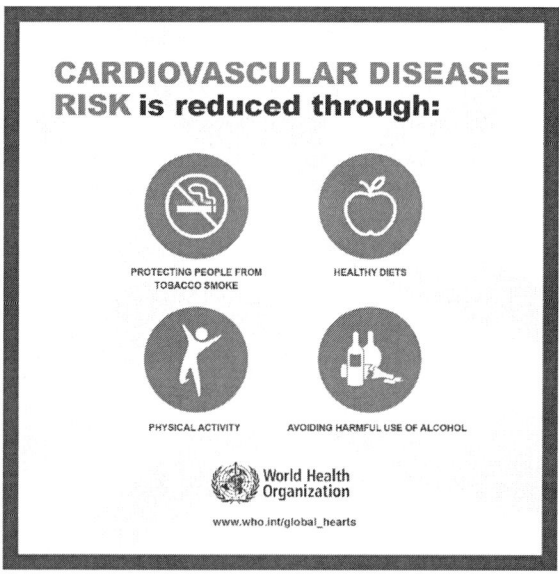

Figure 3. The four main preventive actions advocated by the WHO to reduce CVD risk. Source: https://www.who.int/news-room/fact-sheets/detail/cardiovascular-diseases-(cvds)

What are cardiovascular diseases?
Information by the WHO

'Cardiovascular diseases (CVDs) are a group of disorders of the heart and blood vessels and they include:

- coronary heart disease – disease of the blood vessels supplying the heart muscle
- cerebrovascular disease – disease of the blood vessels supplying the brain
- peripheral arterial disease – disease of blood vessels supplying the arms and legs

- rheumatic heart disease – damage to the heart muscle and heart valves from rheumatic fever, caused by streptococcal bacteria
- congenital heart disease – malformations of heart structure existing at birth
- deep vein thrombosis and pulmonary embolism – blood clots in the leg veins, which can dislodge and move to the brain, heart and lungs

Heart attacks and strokes are usually acute events and are mainly caused by a blockage that prevents blood from flowing to the heart or brain. The most common reason for this is a build-up of fatty deposits on the inner walls of the blood vessels that supply the heart or brain. Strokes can also be caused by bleeding from a blood vessel in the brain or from blood clots.' https://www.who.int/news-room/fact-sheets/detail/cardiovascular-diseases-(cvds)

What are the risk factors for cardiovascular disease?

The most important behavioural risk factors of heart disease and stroke are unhealthy diet, physical inactivity, tobacco use, and harmful use of alcohol. The effects of behavioural risk factors may show up in individuals as raised blood pressure, raised blood glucose, raised blood lipids, and overweight and obesity. These intermediate risks factors can be measured in primary care facilities and indicate an increased risk of developing a heart attack, stroke, heart failure, and other complications.

Cessation of tobacco use, reduction of salt in the diet, increased consumption of fruits and vegetables, regular physical activity, and avoidance of harmful use of alcohol have been shown to reduce the risk of CVD. In addition, drug treatment of diabetes, hypertension, and high blood lipids may be necessary to reduce cardiovascular risk and prevent heart attacks and strokes. Health policies that create conducive environments for making healthy choices affordable and available are important in motivating people to adopt and sustain healthy behaviours.

There are also several underlying determinants of CVDs or the causes of the causes. These are a reflection of the major forces driving social, economic and cultural change – globalization, urbanization, and population ageing. Other determinants of CVDs include poverty, stress, and hereditary factors.

Concluding remarks

A large number of studies exploring the CVD risk by oral infections have been performed worldwide. Most of these studies indicate an increased risk.

References

1. Tonetti, MS, Van Dyke, TE, and Working Group 1 of the Joint EFP/AAP Workshop. 2013. "Periodontitis and Atherosclerotic Cardiovascular Disease: Consensus Report of the Joint EFP/AAP Workshop on Periodontitis and Systemic Diseases." *Journal of Periodontology*, No. 84 (4 Suppl): S24–S29.

2. Buhlin, K. 2004. "The Role of Periodontitis in Cardiovascular Disease." PhD diss., University of Stockholm.

3. Tuomainen, A. 2009. "Inflammation-Induced Atherogenesis, Liver Alterations, and Cardiovascular Outcome." PhD diss., University of Helsinki.

4. Håheim, Lise L, Schwarze, PE, Thelle, DS, Nafstad, P, Rønningen, KS, and Olsen, I. 2020. "Low Levels of Antibodies for the Oral Bacterium *Tannerella forsythia* Predict Cardiovascular Disease Mortality in Men with Myocardial Infarction: A Prospective Cohort Study." *Medical Hypotheses*, No. 138: 109575.

5. Kerrigan, SW, and Cox, D. 2011. "Biological Mechanisms: Platelets and Bacteria – Current Scientific Evidence and Methods of Analyses." In *Oral Infections and Cardiovascular Disease*, edited by Lise L Håheim, 45–66. New York, NY: Bentham Sciences.

6. Genco, R, Offenbacher, S, and Beck, J. 2002. "Periodontal Disease and Cardiovascular Disease: Epidemiology and Possible Mechanisms." *Journal of the American Dental Association*, No. 133 Suppl: 14S–22S.

7. De Stefano, F, Anda, RF, Kahn, HS, Williamson, DF, and Russell, CM. 1993. "Dental Disease and Risk of Coronary Heart Disease and Mortality." *British Medical Journal*, No. 306: 688–691.

8. Mattila, KJ, Valtonen, VV, Nieminen, M, and Huttunen, JK. 1995. "Dental Infection and the Risk of New Coronary Events: Prospective Study of Patients with Documented Coronary Artery Disease." *Clinical Infectious Diseases*, No. 20: 588–592.

9. Joshipura, KJ, Rimm, EB, Douglass, CW, Trichopoulos, D, Ascherio, A, and Willett, WC. 1996. "Poor Oral Health and Coronary Heart Disease." *Journal of Dental Research*, No. 75: 16316.

10.   Beck, J, Garcia, R, Heiss, G, Vokonas, PS, and Offenbacher, S. 1996. "Periodontal Disease and Cardiovascular Disease." *Journal of Periodontology*, No. 67 (10 Suppl): 1123–1137.

11.   Morrison, H, Ellison, L, and Taylor, G. 1999. "Periodontal Disease and Risk of Fatal Coronary Heart and Cerebrovascular Diseases." *Journal of Cardiovascular Risk*, No. 6: 7–11.

12.   Wu, T, Trevisan, M, Genco, RJ, Dorn, JP, Falkner, KL, and Sempos, CT. 2000. "Periodontal Disease and Cerebrovascular Disease: The First National Health and Nutrition Examination Survey and Its Follow-Up Study." *Archives of General Internal Medicine*, No. 160: 2749–2755.

13.   Hujoel, P, Drangsholt, M, Spiekerman, C, and DeRouen, T. 2000. "Periodontal Disease and Coronary Heart Disease Risk." *JAMA*, No. 284: 1406–1410.

14.   Howell, TH, Ridker, PM, Ajani, UA, Hennekens, CH, and Christen, WG. 2001. "Periodontal Disease and Risk of Subsequent Cardiovascular Disease in U.S. Male Physicians." *Journal of the American College of Cardiology*, No. 37: 445–450.

15.   Desvarieux, M, Demmer, RT, Rundek, T, Boden-Albala, B, Jacobs Jr, DR, Papapanou, PN, Sacco, RL, and Oral Infections and Vascular Disease Epidemiology Study (INVEST). 2003. "Relationship between Periodontal Disease, Tooth Loss, and Carotid Artery Plaque: The Oral Infections and Vascular Disease Epidemiology Study (INVEST)." *Stroke*, No. 34: 2120–2125.

16.   Desvarieux, M, Demmer, RT, Jacobs Jr, DR, Rundek, T, Boden-Albala, B, Sacco, RL, and Papapanou, PN. 2010. "Periodontal Bacteria and Hypertension: The Oral Infections and Vascular Disease Epidemiology Study (INVEST)." *Journal of Hypertension*, No. 28: 1413–1421.

17.   Desvarieux, M, Demmer, RT, Rundek, T, Boden-Albala, B, Jacobs Jr, DR, Sacco, RL, and Papapanou, PN. 2005. "Periodontal Microbiota and Carotid Intima-Media Thickness: The Oral Infections and Vascular Disease Epidemiology Study (INVEST)." *Circulation*, No. 111: 576–582.

18.   Yu, YH, Chasman, DI, Buring, JE, Rose, L, and Ridker, PM. 2015. "Cardiovascular Risks Associated with Incident and Prevalent Periodontal Disease." *Journal of Clinical Periodontology*, No. 42: 21–28.

19.   Tuomainen, A, Nyyssönen, K, Laukkanen, JA, Tervahartiala, T, Tuomainen, T-P, Salonen, JT, Sorsa, T, and Pussinen, PJ. 2007. "Serum Matrix Metalloproteinase-8 Concentrations Are Associated

with Cardiovascular Outcome in Men." *Arteriosclerosis, Thrombosis, and Vascular Biology*, No. 27: 2722–2728.

20.   de Oliveira, C, Watt, R, and Hamer, M. 2010. "Toothbrushing, Inflammation, and Risk of Cardiovascular Disease: Results from Scottish Health Survey." *British Medical Journal*, No. 340: c2451. https://doi.org/10.1136/bmj.c2451

21.   Watt, RG, Tsakos, G, de Oliveira, C, and Hamer, M. 2012. "Tooth Loss and Cardiovascular Disease Mortality Risk – Results from the Scottish Health Survey." *PLoS One*, No. 7: e30797.

22.   Liljestrand, JM, Havulinna, AS, Paju, S, Männistö, S, Salomaa, V, and Pussinen, PJ. 2015. "Missing Teeth Predict Incident Cardiovascular Events, Diabetes, and Death." *Journal of Dental Research*, No. 94: 1055–1062.

23.   LaMonte, MJ, Genco, RJ, Hovey, KM, Wallace, RB, Freudenheim, JL, Michaud, DS, Mai, X, Tinker, LF, Salazar, CR, Andrews, CA, Li, W, Eaton, CB, Martin, LW, and Wactawski-Wende, J. 2017. "History of Periodontitis Diagnosis and Edentulism as Predictors of Cardiovascular Disease, Stroke, and Mortality in Postmenopausal Women." *Journal of the American Heart Association*, No. 6: 1-11.

24.   Håheim, Lise L, Nafstad, P, Olsen, I, Schwarze, P, and Rønningen, KS. 2009. "C-reactive Protein Variations for Different Chronic Somatic Disorders." *Scandinavian Journal of Public Health*, No. 37: 640–646.

25.   Almeida, APCPSC, Fagundes, NCF, Maia, LC, Lima, RR. 2018. "Is There an Association between Periodontitis and Atherosclerosis in Adults? A Systematic Review." *Current Vascular Pharmacology*, No. 16: 569–582.

26.   Kolltveit, KM, Geiran, O Tronstad, L, and Olsen, I. 2002. "Multiple Bacteria in Calcific Aortic Valve Stenosis." *Microbial Ecology in Health and Disease*, No. 14 (2): 110–117. https://doi.org/10.1080/08910600260081766

27.   Marques da Silva, R, Lingaas, PS, Geiran, O, Tronstad, L, and Olsen, I. 2003. "Multiple Bacteria in Aortic Aneurysms." *Journal of Vascular Surgery*, No. 38 (6): 1384–1389. https://doi.org/10.1016/s0741-5214(03)00926-1

28.   Müller, HP. 2002. Spielt die marginale Parodontitis eine Rolle in der Pathogenese kardio- und zerebrovaskulärer Erkrankungen? [Does Chronic Periodontitis Play a Role in the Pathogenesis of Cardiovascular and Cerebrovascular Diseases?]. *Gesundheitswesen*, No. 64: 89–98.

29. Blaizot, A, Vergnes, JN, Nuwwareh, S, Amar, J, and Sixou, M. 2009. "Periodontal Diseases and Cardiovascular Events: Meta-analysis of Observational Studies." Int Dent J. 2009; 59:197-209.

30. Larvin, H, Kang, J, Aggarwal, VR, Pavitt, S, and Wu, J. 2021. "Risk of Incident Cardiovascular Disease in People with Periodontal Disease: A Systematic Review and Meta-analysis." *Clinical and Experimental Dental Research*, No. 7: 109–122.

31. Joshi, C, Bapat, R, Anderson, W, Dawson, D, Hijazi, K, and Cherukara, G. 2021. "Detection of Periodontal Microorganisms in Coronary Atheromatous Plaque Specimens of Myocardial Infarction Patients: A Systematic Review and Meta-analysis." *Trends in Cardiovascular Medicine*, No. 31: 69–82.

32. Berlin-Broner, Y, Febbraio, M, and Levin, L. 2017. "Association between Apical Periodontitis and Cardiovascular Diseases: A Systematic Review of the Literature." *International Endodontic Journal*, No. 50: 847–859.

33. D'Aiuto, F, Ready, D, and Tonetti, MS. 2004. "Periodontal Disease and C-reactive Protein-Associated Cardiovascular Risk." *Journal of Periodontal Research*, No. 39: 236–241.

34. Sharma, S, Sridhar, S, McIntosh, A, Messow, C-M, Aguilera, EM, Del Pinto, R, Pietropaoli, D, Gorska, R, Siedlinski, M, Maffia, P, Tomaszewski, M, Guzik, TJ, D'Aiuto, F, and Czesnikiewicz-Guzik, M. 2021. "Periodontal Therapy and Treatment of Hypertension-Alternative to the Pharmacological Approach. A Systematic Review and Meta-analysis." *Pharmacological Research*, No. 166: 105511. https://doi.org/10.1016/j.phrs.2021.105511.

35. Conroy, RM, Pyöälä, K, Fitzgerald, AP, Sans, S, Menotti, A, De Backer, G, De Bacquer, D, Ducimetière, P, Jousilahti, P, Keil, U, Njølstad, I, Oganov, RG, Thomsen, T, Tunstall-Pedoe, H, Tverdal, A, Wedel, H, Whincup, P, Wilhelmsen, L, Graham, IM, and SCORE Project Group. 2003. "Estimation of Ten-Year Risk of Fatal Cardiovascular Disease in Europe: The SCORE Project." *European Heart Journal*, No. 24: 987–1003.

CHAPTER 6

STROKE

Stroke is a rare disease in the young. However, the incidence increases with age, and it is common worldwide. The main specific diagnoses are cerebral infarct, cerebral haemorrhage, cerebral aneurysm, or subarachnoid haemorrhage. The specific diagnosis is best made by imaging techniques (such as MRI or CT scan), in addition to clinical signs and symptoms. Treatment is urgent to prevent further damage to brain functions. The sequela after stroke varies from mild to debilitating paralyses. Because stroke may occur in different areas of the cerebral circulation, the effect on blood flow and the consequences of reduced blood flow presents different symptoms with accompanying paralysis of muscles and organs. Depending on the location of the obstruction in the brain, there is a range of symptoms. One side of the body is suddenly afflicted with loss of motor function of muscles of the face and arm, speech impediment, memory loss, and/or reduced ability to perform daily activities and walking.

The obstruction of cerebral vessels may occur for different reasons, and stroke is a serious disease of the vascular system. A consequence of atherosclerosis is the narrowing of the vessel lumen, causing blood flow obstruction. A common cause of stroke are emboli transported by the circulation. This may be due to heart conditions such as atrial fibrillation (AF), congenital malformations, infectious endocarditis (IE), or dysfunctional valves that form sites were thrombosis may develop and later are released into the circulation and transported to distant sites as emboli. Obstruction of the ascending external carotid artery is a common cause of stroke symptoms and stroke, as well as emboli from the venous part of the circulation.

The WHO reports stroke to be the second most common cause of death in the world after ischaemic heart disease (https://www.who.int/news-room/fact-sheets/detail/the-top-10-causes-of-death) and estimates that about 10% of the world population have chronic periodontitis (https://www.who.int/news-room/fact-sheets/detail/oral-health). It is estimated that oral diseases affect nearly 3.5 billion people. Untreated dental caries (tooth decay) in permanent teeth is the most common health condition, according to the Global Burden of Disease Study 2017 (https://www.who.int/news-room/fact-sheets/detail/oral-health).

According to the WHO, a verified stroke has symptoms lasting more than 24 hours. A stroke that presents with varying intensity of symptoms from a transient paralysis that subsides within 24 hours is called transient ischaemic attack and, according to the WHO definition, is not a stroke. https://www.who.int/healthinfo/statistics/bod_cerebrovasculardiseasestroke.pdf

If oral infections should be associated with or even causal for stroke, is there enough information to explain how this may occur? If there are indications of an association, then treatment of oral infections would be an important prophylactic measure. The high incidence and mortality of stroke has led to many hypotheses regarding causal factors, resultant symptoms, and how to treat them to improve the health of people globally. There are two biologic circulatory mechanisms that are of importance to explore with regard to oral infections – namely, atherosclerosis and thrombosis/emboli.

Epidemiologic research

Oral bacteria in periodontitis are in close proximity to the circulation in the jaw. The bacteria in deep infections are anaerobic, and as they are tissue destructing, they are able to enter the bloodstream and into the vessel walls. The immune system produces antibodies and anti-inflammatory factors (such as CRP and IL-6) to protect against the spread of infection. The level of antibodies varies between individuals, and bacterial products in the circulation may contribute to atherosclerosis and thrombosis. Emboli are formed by the thrombotic effect of blood platelets adhering to each other. Bacteria in the circulation may contribute to the formation of emboli, as they adhere to the platelets. These mechanisms appear to be the main ones and have been explained in Chapter 5.

Several studies have explored the prediction of stroke by examining oral health, including number of remaining teeth, alveolar bone loss, gingivitis, and periodontitis. The number of tooth extractions indicates a high, maybe intermittent, level of dental and/or periodontal infection.

One of the early studies was the first National Health and Nutrition Examination Survey and its follow-up study (1). The study cohort comprised 9,962 participating adults aged 25 to 74 years. The follow-up study concentrated on cerebrovascular accidents. The researchers stratified oral health according to no PD, gingivitis, periodontitis, and edentulousness. ICD-9 codes 430–438 were used to identify nonfatal cases in relevant hospital records and fatal cases by death certificates. In short, the researchers found significant associations between periodontitis, but not gingivitis or edentulousness, and total cerebrovascular accidents (HR = 1.66, 95% CI 1.15–2.39) and nonhaemorrhagic cerebral stroke (HR = 2.11, 95% CI 1.30–3.42). Similar risk levels were seen in the results for White men, White women, and African Americans.

In 2003, results from the large Health Professional Follow-up Study (HPFS) were published about PD and tooth loss as risk factors for ischaemic stroke (2). The participants (N = 51,529) were male health professionals, including dentists, veterinarians, pharmacists, optometrists, osteopaths, and podiatrists. In 1986, they were 40 to 75 years of age. Participants completed mailed questionnaires every two years in a regular follow-up to gain information on changes in medical history, health behaviour, and the occurrence of CVDs and other outcomes. A total of 41,380 men with no history of CVD or diabetes were considered eligible. During the 12 years of follow-up, 349 incident cases of ischaemic stroke identified. Several confounding variables were used in these adjusted analyses, including age, number of cigarettes smoked, obesity, alcohol, exercise, a family history of CVD, multivitamin use, vitamin E use, profession, baseline-reported hypertension, hypercholesterolemia, gender, and socioeconomic status. The researchers found that men with < 25 teeth at the baseline screening had elevated risk compared to men with ≥ 25 teeth (HR = 1.57, 95% CI 1.24–1.98). The association between a history of PD and ischaemic stroke was an HR of 1.33 (95% CI 1.03–1.71).

Another large study is the 14-year prospective follow-up of 867,256 Korean men and women who received health insurance from the National Health Insurance Corporation (3). The participants were medically evaluated between 1992 and 1995, and tooth loss, diabetes, hypertension, and smoking were registered with the aim of studying their independent effects on and interactions with stroke. In that study period, the individuals were aged 30–95 years. The overall prevalence of having one tooth lost was 29.8%, 31.9% for men and 22.3% for women. In the cohort, 28,258 strokes were registered, of which 5,105 were fatal ones. The risk assessed for total stroke in a multivariate model for ≥ 7 teeth lost versus none lost was an HR of 1.3 (95% CI 1.2–1.4) for men and an HR of 1.2 (95% CI 1.0–1.3) for women. For ischaemic and haemorrhagic strokes, the HR values were similar for men and women.

Included in the Physicians' Health Study (N = 22,071) was an RCT of aspirin and beta-carotene, along with a prospective follow-up analysis of 22,037 physicians on the risk of self-reported PD (4). In over 12 years of follow-up, self-reported PD was not found to be an independent predictor for nonfatal stroke, nonfatal MI, or CVD death.

A more precise measure of PD was used in the Veterans Affairs Normative Aging and Dental Longitudinal Study (5). The researchers used radiographs to measure alveolar bone loss and cumulative periodontal probing depth. Data was available for 1,137 dentate men who had dental/medical triannual examinations for up to 34 years (mean 24 years). The researchers found that men aged < 65 years had an increased risk of incident stroke by alveolar bone loss (HR = 5.81, 95% CI 1.63–20.7) but not by probing depth. This association was not observed in older men.

The prospective follow-up of the Oslo II study supports the hypothesis of an association between oral health and the risk of stroke (6, 7). In 2000, 12,764 men were invited for screening, and 6,530 men attended. Oral health data as tooth extraction was self-reported information. Mortality information was given by linkage to the national mortality register. The statistical analyses indicated that for number of tooth extractions > 10, the risk adjusted for known CVD risk factors for cerebral infarct was an HR of 2.92 (95% CI 1.24–6.89). This was independent of the following factors: HDL cholesterol (inversely) (HR = 0.21, 95% CI 0.06–0.76), frequent alcohol consumption (drinking four to seven times per week) (HR = 3.58, 95% CI 1.40–9.13), and diabetes (HR = 4.28, 95% CI 1.68–10.89). The risk factors of mortality for cerebral haemorrhage were age, hs-CRP, and body mass index (BMI) (inversely). For unspecified stroke, age and total cholesterol (inversely) were predictors. Of interest was the observation that the risk factor pattern varied between the specific stroke diagnoses.

Microbiology

Streptococcus mutans is an oral bacterium that causes caries, has a collagen-binding protein (Cnm), and shows platelet aggregation inhibition and MMP-9 activation. Inenaga, Hokamura, Nakano, Nomura et al. analysed whole saliva from 429 hospitalized patients in the period 2010/2011 (8). Included in the study were 48 patients diagnosed with cardioembolic stroke (CES), 151 with non-CES infarct, 54 with intracerebral haemorrhage (ICH), 43 with ruptured intracranial aneurysm, and 97 with unruptured intracranial aneurysm. A total of 79 healthy volunteers were included as a control group. Known CVD risk factors were analysed but not found to be associated with

Cnm rates. The researchers found significant increased high Cnm rates of specific types of *S. mutans* for CES, non-CES, ICH, and ruptured intracranial aneurysm and concluded that further research is needed.

Dental treatment

Invasive dental treatment can reduce infectious loads but is suspected of causing stroke or MI. Chen, D'Aiuto, Yeh, Lai et al. explored this risk using data from a large Taiwanese cohort study of the Taiwanese National Health Care Claim database (9). The authors used two study designs: a) a case-crossover design of 123,819 patients with MI and 327,179 patients with ischaemic stroke and b) a self-controlled study design of 117,655 patients with MI and 298,757 patients with ischaemic stroke. MI risk among those patients without comorbidities was an OR of 1.31 (95% CI 1.08–1.58) for three days and an OR of 1.15 (95% CI 1.01–1.31) for seven days post treatment. At 24 weeks after invasive dental treatment, there were no differences between the groups, and no differences were observed for the ischaemic stroke studies. However, the authors stated that long-term risk cannot be excluded.

Another study from Taiwan was published in 2013 (10). The aim of the study was to investigate if PD treatment would reduce the incidence rate of stroke. In all, 510,762 cases with PD and 208,674 with no PD were included in the period 2000–2010. The cases with PD were categorized as receiving dental prophylaxis, intensive treatment, or no treatment. Ischaemic stroke incidence rate was recorded for the follow-up period. The Cox regression analyses were adjusted for known confounders. The results of the group comparisons for HR of incident stroke risk are as follows:

- ❖ Dental prophylaxis versus non-PD (HR = 0.78, 95% CI 0.75–0.81)
- ❖ Intensive treatment versus non-PD (HR = 0.95, 95% CI 0.91–0.99)
- ❖ PD without treatment versus non-PD in the age group 20–44 years (HR = 1.15, 95% CI 1.07–1.24).
- ❖ PD without treatment versus non-PD (age-stratified analysis) (HR = 2.17, 95% CI 1.64–2.87).

The authors concluded that maintaining oral health by prophylaxis and treatment is important to reduce stroke incidence.

Another relevant study is the 45 and Up Study (New South Wales, Australia) (11). The researchers aimed to investigate oral health and incident hospitalization for ischaemic heart disease (IHD), heart failure

(HF), ischaemic stroke, peripheral vascular disease (PVD), and all-cause mortality. This was a prospective study with a baseline (2006–2009) of 172,630 men of women aged 45–75 years and follow-up until 2011. Oral parameters were tooth loss and self-rated health of teeth and gums. The median follow-up was 3.9 years. Incident hospitalization for IHD, HF, ischaemic stroke, and PVD was 3,239, 212, 283, and 359, and there were 1,908 deaths. All causes, except stroke, increased with increasing tooth loss. Comparing no teeth versus ≥ 20 teeth remaining, the risk for HF was an HR of 1.97 (95% CI 1.27–3.07); for PVD, and HR of 2.53 (95% CI 1.81–3.52); and for all-cause mortality, an HR of 1.60 (95% CI 1.37–1.87).

Atrial fibrillation

Another line of research has been performed in the dental Atherosclerosis Risk in Communities study (12). The researchers studied the association of periodontitis level and dental care utilization with atrial fibrillation (AF) and stroke. At the screening, the degree of periodontitis was stratified as healthy (reference), mild, moderate, and severe. Further, the participants were characterized as regular or episodic dental care users. Using Cox analyses, the researchers tested 17 years of follow-up for AF as a mediator in the periodontitis and stroke association. In all, 5,958 participants were included with no prior history of AF, and 754 were found to have AF during follow-up. Severe PD was found to be associated with AF in the multivariate analysis (HR = 1.31, 95% CI 1.02–1.62). AF was found to mediate the association between severe periodontitis and stroke. The authors made the conclusion that periodontitis is associated with AF and that regular users of dental care had a significantly lower risk of AF observed in the main Atherosclerosis Risk in Communities cohort of 9,666 participants, of whom 1,556 experienced AF during follow-up.

Concluding remarks

The association of oral infections such as gingivitis, periodontitis and tooth loss, or dental treatment with stroke incidence and mortality has been explored in large prospective cohorts worldwide. The observed association between PD and AF risk strengthens the hypothesis of an association between PD and stroke.

References

1.   Wu, T, Trevisan, M, Genco, RJ, Dorn, JP, Falkner, KL, and Sempos, CT. 2000. "Periodontal Disease and Risk of Cerebrovascular Disease: The First National Health and Nutrition Examination Survey and Its Follow-Up Study." *Archives of Internal Medicine*, No. 160: 2749–2755.

2.   Joshipura, KJ, Hung, HC, Rimm, EB, Willett, WC, and Ascherio, Alberto. 2003. "Periodontal Disease, Tooth Loss and Incidence of Ischemic Stroke." *Stroke*, No. 34: 47–52.

3.   Choe, H, Kim, YH, Park, JW, Kim, SY, Lee, S-L, and Jee, SH. 2009. "Tooth Loss, Hypertension and Risk for Stroke in a Korean Population." *Atherosclerosis*, No. 203: 550–556.

4.   Howell, TH, Ridker, PM, Ajani, UA, Hennekens, CH, and Christen, WG. 2001. "Periodontal Disease and Risk of Subsequent Cardiovascular Disease in U.S. Male Physicians." *Journal of the American College of Cardiology*, No. 37: 445–450.

5.   Jimenez, M, Krall, EA, Garcia, RI, Vokonas, PS, and Dietrich, T. 2009. "Periodontitis and Incidence of Cerebrovascular Disease in Men." *Annals of Neurology*, No. 66: 505–512.

6.   Håheim, Lise L, Rønningen, KS, Nafstad, P, Schwarze, PE, Thelle, DS, and Olsen, I. 2017. "Number of Tooth Extractions Is Associated with Increased Risk of Mortality." *SciTz Dentistry: Research & Therapy*, No. 2 (1).

7.   Håheim, Lise L, Nafstad, Per, Schwarze, Per E, Olsen, Ingar, Rønningen, Kjersti S, and Thelle, Dag S. 2019. "Oral Health and Cardiovascular Disease Risk Factors and Mortality of Cerebral Haemorrhage, Cerebral Infarction and Unspecified Stroke in Elderly Men: A Prospective Cohort Study." *Scandinavian Journal of Public Health*, No. 48: 762–769. https://doi.org/10.1177/1403494819879351

8.   Inenaga, C, Hokamura, K, Nakano, K, Nomura, R, Naka, S, Ohashi, T, Ooshima, T, Kuriyama, N, Hamasaki, T, Wada, K, Umemura, K, and Tanaka, T. 2018. "A Potential New Risk Factor for Stroke: *Streptococcus mutans* with Collagen-Binding Protein." *World Neurosurgery*, No. 113: e77–e81.

9.   Chen, TT, D'Aiuto, F, Yeh, YC, Lai, MS, Chien, KL, and Tu, YK. 2019. "Risk of Myocardial Infarction and Ischemic Stroke after Dental Treatments." *Journal of Dental Research*, No. 98: 157–163. https://doi.org/10.1177/0022034518805745

10.   Lee, YL, Hu, HY, Huang, N, Hwang, DK, Chou, P, and Chu, D. 2013. "Dental Prophylaxis and Periodontal Treatment Are Protective Factors to Ischemic Stroke." *Stroke*, No. 44: 1026–1030.

11.   Joshy, G, Arora, M, Korda, RJ, Chalmers, J, and Banks, E. 2016. "Is Poor Oral Health a Risk Marker for incident Cardiovascular Disease Hospitalisation and All-Cause Mortality? Findings from 172 630 Participants from the Prospective 45 and Up Study." BMJ Open. 2016; 6: e012386.

12.   Sen, S, Redd, K, Trivedi, T, Moss, K, Alonso, A, Soliman, EZ, Magnani, JW, Chen, LY, Gottesman, RF, Rosamond, W, Beck, J, and Offenbacher, S. 2021. "Periodontal Disease, Atrial Fibrillation and Stroke." *American Heart Journal*, No. 235: 36–43.

CHAPTER 7

PERIPHERAL ARTERIAL DISEASE

Scientific evidence

Three recent SRs, as well as a large single study, have been identified and are reported here.

Chinese researchers sought to evaluate the association between PD and peripheral arterial disease (PAD) (1). Seven studies, including a total of 4,307 participants, were included in the meta-analysis, and the effect measure was weighted mean difference (WMD) and 95% CIs. The researchers compared periodontitis risk in patients diagnosed with PAD versus patients without PAD. The pooled analysis showed a significant difference (RR = 1.70, 95% CI 1.25–2.29, p = 0.01). Number of missing teeth were significantly different between the two groups (WMD = 3.75, 95% CI 1.31–6.19, p = 0.003) but not for clinical attachment loss (CAL).

German researchers studied the association of PD with peripheral arterial occlusive disease (PAOD) (2). In their SR, they detected 755 studies, and 17 were included in a qualitative analysis. An association between PD and PAOD was observed, and two studies reported an association between tooth loss and PAOD. Six studies examined the pathology involved. None of the studies were negative for an association. In four large cohorts, the risk estimates ranged from 1.3 to 3.9, adjusted for known CVD risk factors.

Another Chinese SR investigated the association of PD with specific PAD disorders (3). The researchers included 25 studies (a total of 22,090 participants). The overall study results of the meta-analysis was heterogenic, as shown by $I^2 = 80.5\%$ (OR = 1.60, 95% CI 1.41–1.82, p < 0.001). The results of the subgroup analyses were as follows: lower extremity arterial disease (OR = 3.00, 95% CI 2.23–4.04, p < 0.001, $I^2 =$ 0%) and carotid artery disease (OR = 1.39, 95% CI 1.24–1.56, p < 0.001, $I^2 =$ 79.4%).

A large single study is worth mentioning – the Health Professionals Follow-up Study (HPFS), an American study published in 2003 (4). This was a prospective study of 45,136 men free of CVD at baseline. After a 12-year follow-up, the researchers identified 342 cases of PAD. The researchers used different oral disease measurements and estimated the PAD risk during follow-up. Number of teeth at baseline did not predict PAD, but incident tooth loss did, (RR = 1.39, 95% CI 1.07–1.82). The RR of history of PD was 1.41 (95% CI 1.12–1.77), with the analyses adjusted for known CVD risk factors. Tooth loss related to a history of PD was further examined; if a history of PD was reported, then subsequent tooth loss showed an RR of 1.88 (95% CI 1.27–2.77). No association was observed among men without prior history of PD. Previous tooth loss two to six years prior to screening predicted PAD.

Concluding remarks

The studies mentioned in this chapter involved different risks of exposure from a history of PD, current PD, and tooth extractions before screening or during follow-up. Although the meta-analyses show heterogeneity, the sum of the results draw in the same direction of elevated PAD risk due to PD.

References

1. Yang, S, Zhao, LS, Cai, C, Shi, Q, Wen, N, and Xu, J. 2018. "Association between Periodontitis and Peripheral Artery Disease: A Systematic Review and Meta-analysis." *BMC Cardiovascular Disorders*, No. 18 (1): 141. https://doi.org/10.1186/s12872-018-0879-0

2. Kaschwich, M, Behrendt, CA, Heydecke, G, Bayer, A, Debus, ES, Seedorf, U, and Aarabi, G. 2019. "The Association of Periodontitis and Peripheral Arterial Occlusive Disease—A Systematic Review." *International Journal of Molecular Sciences*, No. 20 (12): 2936. https://doi.org/10.3390/ijms20122936

3. Wang, J, Geng, X, Sun, J, Zhang, S, Yu, W, Zhang, X, and Liu, H. 2019. "The Risk of Periodontitis for Peripheral Vascular Disease: A Systematic Review." *Reviews in Cardiovascular Medicine*, No. 20 (2): 81–89. https://doi.org/10.31083/j.rcm.2019.02.52

4. Hung, HC, Willett, W, Merchant, A, Rosner, BA, Ascherio, A, and Joshipura, KJ. 2003. "Oral Health and Peripheral Arterial Disease." *Circulation*, No. 107 (8): 1152–1157. https://doi.org/10.1161/01.cir.0000051456.68470.c8

CHAPTER 8

INFECTIVE ENDOCARDITIS

Dental work often involves bleeding as part of the treatment of, for example, gingivitis and periodontitis; the positioning of implants; tooth extractions; oral surgery; and examinations. Consequently, dentists are concerned about the spread of infection to the heart, and one concern is the potential to cause infective endocarditis (IE) in patients at risk of systemic disease, giving rise to damage to the heart valves. IE is a rare but serious disease with a high degree of morbidity, require long courses of antibiotic treatment, and has a high fatality rate. Direct factors of IE are difficult to establish, but a vulnerable cardiac lining (endothelium) and a high load of oral bacteria appear to be part of the causal picture. It has been established that the microorganisms involved are mainly viridans streptococci, enterococci, coagulase-positive staphylococci or coagulase-negative staphylococci (1). Oral streptococci belong to the viridans group of bacteria (*Streptococcus mutans* and *S. sanguis*). These are usually part of the oral microbiome/plaque attached to the different surfaces in the mouth. As they develop infections, these bacteria may enter the bloodstream and be dispersed to distant organs, such as the heart. Tooth brushing with gingival bleeding is believed to be a part of this process but was not shown in patients with gingivitis compared to healthy individuals in research study (2, 3).

IE treatment involves systemic antibiotics for four to six weeks and sometimes replacement of damaged heart valves need to be performed. Consequently, this has involved giving a short course of prophylactic antibiotics to patients considered to be at risk for IE. Much concern has also risen about the possible unnecessary use of antibiotics, as it increases the risk of infections with antibiotic-resistant bacteria and this limits treatment options. Extensive research has been performed, but more knowledge is needed to fully understand the systemic and immunologic pathology of the spread of infections and the following tissue damage in, for example, IE (4). Oral bacteria or bacterial DNA have been identified in histopathologic studies of stenotic heart valves and aneurysms of the descending aorta, confirming the invasive ability of oral and other bacteria (5, 6).

Descriptive studies

A retrospective study from Alabama, US, from 1981 provided results of patients with bacterial endocarditis and their history of dental care and bacteraemia in the period 1969–1979 (7). The researchers found that 16% of persons with bacterial endocarditis had a history of recent dental care or pathology. They also found that *Streptococcus viridans* was the predominant bacterium of bacterial endocarditis. Patients with prosthetic heart valves had the highest mortality rate. Chronic heart valve disease posed a high risk, as well as dental infections such as PD and teeth abscesses.

A particular vulnerable group is children with congenital heart disease (8). Nosrati, Eckert, Kowolik, Ho et al. showed in a case-control study that children with cardiac conditions have a higher prevalence of PD, evidenced by gingivitis, plaque, and calculus. These children need a regular follow-up on their periodontal status.

A Brazilian study investigated if there was an increased risk for pregnant women with rheumatic fever versus healthy pregnant women with regard to oral health (9). Clinical and microbiologic oral health examinations were performed. The researchers concluded that clinical and microbiological status was comparable between both groups of women.

Prevalence

Šutej, Peroš, Trkulja, Rudež et al. conducted a retrospective survey of patients with IE in Croatia to assess to what degree the cases were odontogenic or not (10). Among 386 patients, 68 cases were confirmed as odontogenic IE, and 318 patients with IE of other origin. The diagnosis of odontogenic IE was based on two separate bacterial cultures showing exclusive oral pathogens of odontogenic bacterial cultures or *S. viridans* associated with previous or recent dental treatment. Dental procedure previous to IE did not occur in 91.2% of the cases. In all, 47.1% had a previous cardiac condition, increasing their IE risk.

Ninomiya, Hashimoto, Yamanouchi, Fukumura et al. conducted a cross-sectional study of 119 patients with periodontitis, where 78 had valvular heart disease (VHD) (11). The researchers found that patients with VHD had poorer oral health than patients without VHD in terms of number of tooth extractions and alveolar bone loss. The bacterial status was different, as Pg IgG titer > 1.68 and Pg fimA type II genotype was highest in patients with IE.

From the Italian Registry of Infective Endocarditis, Chirillo, Faggiano, Cecconi, Moreo et al. reported about patients enrolled between 2007 and 2010 (12). The aim of the researchers was to evaluate the use of prophylactic antibiotics in patients with a cardiac condition who require an intervention. They studied 677 patients, mainly men with IE, and half had predisposing cardiac conditions. The researchers observed that nondental procedures (n = 139) were performed more often in these patients than dental procedures (n = 32), and therefore, prophylactic antibiotics for preventing IE would yield less cases of IE after dental procedures. *S. aureus* was the most common causative bacteria for IE. *S. viridans* was isolated from patients who had undergone prior dental care. Preoperative prophylactic antibiotics was given to seven patients. Surgical and hospital mortality was greatest in the nondental procedures group.

Prophylactic dental treatment

In a study from Taiwan, Chen, Liu, Chao, Wang et al. identified 736 patients with newly diagnosed IE in the National Health Insurance Research Database in the period 2000–2009 (13). For each patient, 10 controls were enrolled in the study. The controls were matched on age, sex, and underlying diseases. The cases and controls were compared with regard to dental scaling before being included in the study. The controls had dental scaling more often than the cases. The researchers found a borderline significant difference with dental scaling once in two years reducing the risk by 15% (OR = 0.85, 95% CI 0.69–1.01, p = 0.058). Patients who did dental scaling twice a year had a significant reduced risk (OR = 0.70, 95% CI 0.54–0.89, p = 0.005).

Bratel, Kennergren, Dernevik, and Hakeberg from Sweden sought to evaluate the importance of prophylactic dental treatment to prevent and remove infections before heart valve surgery, and they followed participants for 16 years on the incidence of IE (14). They studied patients with three to six months of dental treatment (n = 149) versus a control group of no prophylactic treatment (n = 103), and all patients were to undergo heart valve surgery. The investigators found that 37% of patients in the study group survived versus 45% in the control group. The authors concluded that they did not find that dental treatment before heart valve surgery improved survival.

Guidelines for the use of prophylactic antibiotics

Since 1955, the American Heart Association (AHA) has developed guidelines on antibiotic prophylaxis (AP) to prevent IE, including medical and dental treatment and other types of interventions. In their 2007 revision, they decided to limit the conditions for which AP was considered an important option (15). Research had established that IE could occur after dental treatment but was less common than previously thought. In addition, studies on the effect of AP in randomized controlled trials had not been done, as IE is a rare condition and the studies need a long follow-up. The AHA concluded as follows:

'The major changes in the updated recommendations include the following: (1) The Committee concluded that only an extremely small number of cases of infective endocarditis might be prevented by antibiotic prophylaxis for dental procedures, even if such prophylactic therapy were 100% effective. (2) Infective endocarditis prophylaxis for dental procedures is reasonable only for patients with underlying cardiac conditions associated with the highest risk of adverse outcome from infective endocarditis. (3) For patients with these underlying cardiac conditions, prophylaxis is reasonable for all dental procedures that involve manipulation of gingival tissue or the periapical region of teeth or perforation of the oral mucosa. (4) Prophylaxis is not recommended based solely on an increased lifetime risk of acquisition of infective endocarditis. (5) Administration of antibiotics solely to prevent endocarditis is not recommended for patients who undergo a genitourinary or gastrointestinal tract procedure. These changes are intended to define more clearly when infective endocarditis prophylaxis is or is not recommended and to provide more uniform and consistent global recommendations'.

In 2012, Canadian researchers reported that from 2001 to 2010, there was a 3% yearly decrease in IE in Canada (16). The introduction of the AHA guidelines in Canada did not make an impact on incidence.

In 2015, the ESC published its revised guidelines for IE management. Regarding IE prevention as a consequence of dental treatment, their recommendation was not to use prophylactic antibiotics for a wide range of dental treatments. The reason being that mild bacteraemia arises after everyday tooth brushing and the chewing of food. The revised 2015 guideline (Table 3) defines which patients are at risk of bacteraemia in high-risk procedures and for whom AP can be considered (17):

'Cardiac conditions at highest risk of infective endocarditis for which prophylaxis should be considered when a high-risk procedure is performed.

Recommendations: Antibiotic prophylaxis should be considered for patients at highest risk for IE:

(1) Patients with any prosthetic valve, including a transcatheter valve, or those in whom any prosthetic material was used for cardiac valve repair.
(2) Patients with a previous episode of IE.
(3) Patients with CHD:
    (a) Any type of cyanotic CHD.
    (b) Any type of CHD repaired with a prosthetic material, whether placed surgically or by percutaneous techniques, up to 6 months after the procedure or lifelong if residual shunt or valvular regurgitation remains.

Antibiotic prophylaxis is not recommended in other forms of valvular or CHD'.

The UK National Institute for Health and Care Excellence (NICE) issued a guideline in 2008, with an update in 2016 (18). They conducted an SR of the literature regarding the effect of AP on IE. As they found no studies according to their inclusion criteria, they concluded there was no evidence for AP preventing IE related to interventions, dental or other, and did not recommend AP. This was controversial in comparison to AHA and ESC guidelines. The consequence of this practice is later demonstrated in the reduced prescription of prophylactic antibiotics and, ultimately, a rise of IE incidence in the UK (19). NICE have not changed their guidance. Data from English hospitals indicate a large change (86% rise) from the stable incidence in 1998/1999 to 2009/2010 of 26.6 cases per million inhabitants to 50.0 cases per million inhabitants in 2018/2019 (20).

Concluding remarks

How does one understand and use the available scientific evidence of all levels of study designs? Clinical (medical/dental) trials are exposed to ethical dilemmas. IE is rare, and relevant randomized trials of good quality have not been performed. It should be noted that there has never been an RCT on tobacco smoking and the associated risk of cancer or CVD. Likewise, it would be unethical to perform another randomized study regarding high sugar levels in the diet and the associated possible risk of dental caries, as one study has been performed.

References

1.   Giessel BE, Koenig CE, and Blake RL. 2000. "Management of bacterial Endocarditis." *American Family Physician*. 61 (6): 1725-1732.

2.   Lockhart, PB, Brennan, MT, Thornhill, M, Michalowicz, BS, Noll, J, Bahrani-Mougeot, FK, and Sasser, HC. 2009. "Poor Oral Hygiene as a Risk Factor for Infective Endocarditis-Related Bacteremia." *Journal of the American Dental Association*, No. 140 (10): 1238–1244. https://doi.org/10.14219/jada.archive.2009.0046

3.   Hartzell, JD, Torres, D, Kim, P, and Wortmann, G. 2005. "Incidence of Bacteremia after Routine Tooth Brushing." *American Journal of the Medical Sciences*, No. 329 (4): 178–180. https://doi.org/10.1097/00000441-200504000-00003

4.   Pizzo, G, Guiglia, R, Lo Russo, L, and Campisi, G. 2010. "Dentistry and Internal Medicine: From the Focal Infection Theory to the Periodontal Medicine Concept." *European Journal of Internal Medicine*, No. 21 (6): 496–502. https://doi.org/10.1016/j.ejim.2010.07.011

5.   Kolltveit, KM, Geiran, O Tronstad, L, and Olsen, I. 2002. "Multiple Bacteria in Calcific Aortic Valve Stenosis." *Microbial Ecology in Health and Disease*, No. 14 (2): 110–117. https://doi.org/10.1080/08910600260081766

6.   Marques da Silva, R, Lingaas, PS, Geiran, O, Tronstad, L, and Olsen, I. 2003. "Multiple Bacteria in Aortic Aneurysms." *Journal of Vascular Surgery*, No. 38 (6): 1384–1389. https://doi.org/10.1016/s0741-5214(03)00926-1

7.   Thornton, JB, and Alves, JC. 1981. "Bacterial Endocarditis. A Retrospective Study of Cases Admitted to the University of Alabama Hospitals from 1969 to 1979." *Oral Surgery, Oral Medicine, Oral Pathology, and Oral Radiology*, No. 52 (4): 379–383. https://doi.org/10.1016/0030-4220(81)90334-0

8.   Nosrati, E, Eckert, GJ, Kowolik, MJ, Ho, JG, Schamberger, MS, and Kowolik, JE. 2013. "Gingival Evaluation of the Pediatric Cardiac Patient." *Pediatric Dentistry*, No. 35 (5): 456–462.

9.   Avila, WS, Timerman, L, Romito, GA, Marcelino, SL, Neves, IL, Zugaib, M, and Grinberg, M. 2011. "Periodontal Disease in Pregnant Patients with Rheumatic Valvular Disease: Clinical and Microbiological Study." *Arquivos Brasileiros de Cardiologia*, No. 96 (4): 307–311. https://doi.org/10.1590/s0066-782x2011005000034.

10. Šutej, I, Peroš, K, Trkulja, V, Rudež, I, Barić, D, Alajbeg, I, Pintarić, H, Stevanović, R, and Lepur, D. 2020. "The Epidemiological and Clinical Features of Odontogenic Infective Endocarditis." *European Journal of Clinical Microbiology & Infectious Diseases*, No. 39 (4): 637–645. https://doi.org/10.1007/s10096-019-03766-x

11. Ninomiya, M, Hashimoto, M, Yamanouchi, K, Fukumura, Y, Nagata, T, and Naruishi, K. 2020. "Relationship of Oral Conditions to the Incidence of Infective Endocarditis in Periodontitis Patients with Valvular Heart Disease: A Cross-Sectional Study." *Clinical Oral Investigations*, No. 24 (2): 833–840. https://doi.org/10.1007/s00784-019-02973-2

12. Chirillo, F, Faggiano, P, Cecconi, M, Moreo, A, Squeri, A, Gaddi, O, Cecchi, E, and Italian Registry on Infective Endocarditis (RIEI) Investigators. 2016. "Predisposing Cardiac Conditions, Interventional Procedures, and Antibiotic Prophylaxis among Patients with Infective Endocarditis." *American Heart Journal*, No. 179: 42–50. https://doi.org/10.1016/j.ahj.2016.03.028

13. Chen, SJ, Liu, CJ, Chao, TF, Wang, KL, Wang, FD, Chen, TJ, and Chiang, CE. 2013. "Dental Scaling and Risk Reduction in Infective Endocarditis: A Nationwide Population-Based Case-Control Study." *Canadian Journal of Cardiology*, No. 29 (4): 429–433. https://doi.org/10.1016/j.cjca.2012.04.018

14. Bratel, J, Kennergren, C, Dernevik, L, and Hakeberg, M. 2011. "Treatment of Oral Infections Prior to Heart Valve Surgery Does Not Improve Long-Term Survival." *Swedish Dental Journal*, No. 35 (2): 49–55.

15. Wilson, W, Taubert, KA, Gewitz, M, Lockhart, PB, Baddour, LM, Levison, M, Bolger, A, Cabell, CH, Takahashi, M, Baltimore, RS, Newburger, JW, Strom, BL, Tani, LY, Gerber, M, Bonow, RO, Pallasch, T, Shulman, ST, Rowley, AH, Burns, JC, Ferrieri, P, Gardner, T, Goff, D, Durack, DT, Council on Scientific Affairs of the American Dental Association, American Academy of Pediatrics, Infectious Diseases Society of America, International Society of Chemotherapy for Infection and Cancer, and Pediatric Infectious Diseases Society. 2007. "Prevention of Infective Endocarditis. Guidelines from the American Heart Association: A Guideline from the American Heart Association Rheumatic Fever, Endocarditis, and Kawasaki Disease Committee, Council on Cardiovascular Disease in the Young, and the Council on Clinical Cardiology, Council on Cardiovascular Surgery and Anesthesia, and the Quality of Care and

Outcomes Research Interdisciplinary Working Group." *Circulation*, No. 116: 1736–1754 https://doi.org/10.1161/CIRCULATIONAHA.106.183095

16.   Mackie, AS, Liu, W, Marelli, AJ, and Kaul, P. 2012. "The Incidence of Endocarditis in Canada Is Decreasing." *Circulation*, No. 126: A17637.

17.   Habib, G, Lancellotti, P, Antunes, MJ, Bongiorni, MG, Casalta, J-P, Del Zotti, F, Dulgheru, R, El Khoury, G, Erba, PA, Iung, B, Miro, JM, Mulder, BJ, Plonska-Gosciniak, E, Price, S, Roos-Hesselink, J, Snygg-Martin, U, Thuny, F, Mas, PT, Vilacosta, I, Zamorano, JL, and European Society of Cardiology Scientific Document Group. 2015. "2015 ESC Guidelines for the Management of Infective Endocarditis: The Task Force for the Management of Infective Endocarditis of the European Society of Cardiology (ESC). Endorsed by: European Association for Cardio-Thoracic Surgery (EACTS), the European Association of Nuclear Medicine (EANM)." *European Heart Journal*, No. 36 (44): 3075–3128. https://doi.org/10.1093/eurheartj/ehv319

18.   National Institute for Health and Care Excellence. July 2016. "Prophylaxis against Infective Endocarditis: Antimicrobial Prophylaxis against Infective Endocarditis in Adults and Children Undergoing Interventional Procedures." https://www.nice.org.uk/guidance/cg64/chapter/Recommendations Accessed: 15. September 2021

19.   Dayer, MJ, Jones, S, Prendergast, B, Baddour, LM, Lockhart, PB, and Thornhill, MH. 2015. "Incidence of Infective Endocarditis in England, 2000–13: A Secular Trend, Interrupted Time-Series Analysis." *Lancet*, No. 385: 1219–1228.

20.   Thornhill, MH, Dayer, MJ, Nicholl, J, Prendergast, BD, Lockhart, PB, and Baddour, LM. 2020. "An Alarming Rise in Incidence of Infective Endocarditis in England since 2009: Why?" *Lancet*, 395 (10233): 1325-1327. https://doi.org/10.1016/S0140-6736(20)30530-4

CHAPTER 9

DIABETES MELLITUS

Diabetes, a common disorder among people worldwide, is distinguished as two types: type 1 (insulin-dependent) DM, which is mostly common in young persons, and type 2 (noninsulin-dependent) DM, which occurs in adults. Type 2 DM has become more prevalent and is a major health problem, as it is associated with obesity, elevated blood pressure, an unfavourable lipid profile, inactivity, and other factors (including increased risk of heart disease). Metabolic syndrome is considered a precursor state of DM and is defined by increased blood pressure, high blood sugar, excess body fat around the waist, and abnormal cholesterol or triglyceride levels. There is increasing evidence for type 2 diabetes being a chronic inflammation of the pancreas (1). Type 1 diabetes is an autoimmune disorder where the islets of Langerhans in the pancreas are damaged resulting in insulin deficiency and hyperglycaemia (1). Inflammation is emerging as a pathogenic factor in diabetes.

A large number of studies on PD and DM have been performed, and the latest SRs are reported here. Because much has been written about the association between periodontitis and diabetes, it is of interest to know the prevalence of undiagnosed diabetes and prediabetes in patients attending dental clinics. Nine studies were found eligible, and the results showed a sizeable proportion of patients, depending on the patient population (2). Patients at risk for hyperglycaemia in dental clinic patients were 32.5% using a random blood glucose test and 40.1% after a HbA1c test. Undiagnosed diabetes was estimated to 11.2% and prediabetes 47.4% in the studies.

Oral manifestations

Patients with diabetes may have a specific oral health profile. An SR of the results from 4 longitudinal studies and 15 cross-sectional studies, including a total of 3,712 patients (2,084 with diabetes), showed that PD, periapical lesions, xerostomia (dry mouth), and taste disturbance were more prevalent among DM patients (3). Mauri-Obradors, Estrugo-Devesa, Jané-Salas,

Viñas et al. also found an association between caries and mucosal lesions. Liu, Gkranias, Farias, Spratt et al. reviewed studies and found differences in the oral subgingival microbiota in persons with chronic periodontitis, comparing persons with DM and persons without DM (4). From the five identified relevant studies, the authors could conclude that a low level of the bacterium *Tannerella forsythia* was reported more frequently in persons with DM than in persons without DM. Weaker associations were found for *Porphyromonas gingivalis* and *Actinomyces actinomycetemcomitans*. These and other bacteria are common in chronic periodontitis.

The bidirectional relationship between type 2 diabetes and periodontitis

In 2013, the EFP and the AAP published an SR, with an update in 2018, on the association of diabetes with periodontitis (5, 6). Although they report heterogeneity in this research, they report on a bidirectional relationship. They observed that healthy persons with periodontitis have poor glycaemic control and a high risk of developing DM. They also reported that persons with DM more often have periodontitis and diabetes-related complications. Despite a high number of studies, there still remains more work to be done to explore the heterogeneity of the results on the association between diabetes and periodontitis. The bidirectional relationship between diabetes and chronic periodontitis has been investigated in several studies of varying design and study sample size and including different parameters for periodontitis and diabetes. This has made it difficult to obtain clear and concise results.

Diabetes → periodontitis

In studying whether poorly controlled diabetes is associated with the onset or progression of chronic periodontitis, Nascimento, Leite, Vestergaard, Scheutz et al. investigated the effect of hyperglycaemia and summarised over 13 studies involving a total of 49,262 individuals, including 3,197 diagnosed with diabetes (7). The adjusted estimates of the meta-analyses indicated that diabetes increased the risk of incidence or progression of periodontitis by 86% (RR = 1.86, 95% CI 1.3–2.8). This confirms previous findings of an earlier SR by Ryan, Carnu, and Kamer in 2003 (8). Wu, Yuan, Liu, Li et al. studied this bidirectional relationship with 53 observational studies for meta-analyses of different parameters (9). Among persons with DM, there was an elevated risk of periodontitis (OR = 1.58, p = 0.000) compared to those without DM in 53 observational studies. An elevated periodontitis risk of 34% (p = 0.002) was shown in the cohort studies. Patients with DM had a worse periodontal status, with deeper periodontal pockets, greater attachment loss, and about two more teeth lost than those without DM. This difference may be a result of the reduced glycaemic control of DM.

Periodontitis → diabetes

How common is DM in persons diagnosed with periodontitis? Wu, Yuan, Liu, Li et al. reported the risk of DM in persons with periodontitis of 4.04 (p = 0.000) (9). The researchers showed that severe periodontitis increased the incidence of DM by 53% (p = 0.000). Mild periodontitis had a lesser impact of 28% (p = 0.007). Further, Ziukaite, Slot, and Van der Weijden summarized the results in an SR based on 27 papers (10). The authors found the prevalence of DM in persons with periodontitis to be 13.1% and 9.6% in persons without periodontitis. They found differences between geographical areas as the prevalence of DM in persons with periodontitis was highest in Asian countries (17.1%) and lowest in European countries (4.3%). The overall OR for DM in persons with periodontitis as compared to those without periodontitis was 2.27 (95% CI 1.90–2.72). Due to the studies being performed in many different countries, there was some heterogeneity in the results. The authors reported that self-reported diabetes underestimates the prevalence compared to DM being diagnosed clinically.

An SR of 17 included studies focussed on observational studies such as prospective cohorts and cross-sectional studies to obtain important prospective information (11). The authors found "a small body" of evidence that supports the adverse effect of PD on glycaemic control, diabetes complications, and the development of type 2 (and possibly gestational) diabetes. The authors concluded from this limited and heterogenous evidence that more and larger studies with consistent disease parameters across the studies are warranted. Tooth extractions, considered an indicator of advanced periodontitis, and diabetes have been found to be independent predictors of mortality in men during a 12.5-year follow-up (12).

Periodontal treatment and glycaemic control

Several SRs have been performed, and a chronological presentation is provided in this section. In their Cochrane review from 2015, Simpson, Weldon, Worthington, Needleman et al. evaluated RCTs for two comparisons: 1. Periodontal treatment versus none using 14 studies with

1,499 participants – mean HbA1c was 0.29% lower (95% CI 0.48 lower to 0.10 lower) three to four months posttreatment but 0.02% lower after six months (95% CI 0.20% lower to 0.16% higher). 2. One kind of periodontal treatment compared to different comparative treatments were examined in 21 studies with 920 participants (13). The researchers pooled results of scaling and root planing (SRP) with or without antibiotics and found no consistent effect. Periodontal indicators/measurements as bleeding on probing (BOP), reduction in alveolar height, gingival index (GI), periodontal index, and progressive PD all improved after three to four months in 12 studies and after six months in five studies.

Antibiotic use in addition to SRP was identified in 18 studies of the SR by Santos, Lira-Junior, Fischer, Santos et al. (14). The minimum follow-up of treatment was six months. They found that using systemic antibiotics supplementing standard treatment in the treatment of periodontitis in patients with DM gave a small benefit in PD and BOP. There was no significant effect on clinical attachment level and plaque index (PI) reduction. None of these studies reported on tooth loss or oral health–related gain.

Mauri-Obradors, Jané-Salas, Sabater-Recolons Mdel, Viñas et al., in their SR, investigated the evidence of periodontal treatment lowering HbA1c (15). In 14 of the 21 studies, there was a significant decrease in HbA1c, but there was no decrease in the remaining seven studies.

Botero, Rodríguez, and Agudelo-Suarez summarized the results in an umbrella review of SRs (16). The summary effect over 13 SRs from 1995 to 2015 was a reduction in HbA1c level at three months after intervention, significant in 10 of 12 SRs. However, the effect over a longer follow-up was not shown.

Pérez-Losada, Jané-Salas, Sabater-Recolons, Estrugo-Devesa et al. narrowed their literature search to the period 2013–2015 and identified 13 relevant trials with 1,912 participants (17). The periodontal treatment included radicular curettage and root planing with or without antibiotics. Three of the studies had less than 40 participants included. Seven of the studies showed a significant reduction in HbA1c, but the other six studies did not. The follow-up period after treatment varied between the studies from 3 to 12 months. The authors concluded that treatment improved the periodontal condition, but not all studies showed an improvement in glycaemic control in the persons with type 2 diabetes.

Baeza Hasuike, Iguchi, Suzuki, Kawano et al. concentrated on the treatment of periodontitis by SRP (18). They identified 9 RCTs and found that SRP was statistically significant in reducing HbA1c and CRP. Heterogeneity was not observed between the studies. The conclusion was that SRP treatment has an impact on the metabolic control of diabetes and the systematic inflammation in patients with diabetes.

Adjunctive laser use versus antimicrobial photodynamic therapy (aPDT) to improve HbA1c was assessed in six studies for the SR by Abduljabbar, Javed, Shah, Samer et al. (19). They concluded there is weak scientific evidence for these adjunctive treatments in patients with periodontitis and DM in improving clinical periodontal and glycaemic control in these patients.

Cao, Li, Wu, Yao et al. identified 14 RCTs that compared standard SRP treatment with SRP + additional treatment (20). The authors explored studies that used antibiotic therapy, aPDT, and doxycycline (Doxy) and found that the combination of SRP + aPDT and Doxy ranked best in improving the HbA1c level, but fasting plasma glucose did not improve. Yap and Pulikkotil examined SRP versus SRP + Doxy and, based on six studies, found the addition of Doxy to be ineffective in improving glycaemic control (21).

In 2020, Morales, Cisterna, Cavalla, Jara et al. published an SR with meta-analyses of RCTs of the association of periodontal treatment as SRP with glycaemic control in type 2 diabetes by HbA1c and inflammation by CRP (22). The Medline and Cochrane databases were searched until July 2018, and 349 titles and abstracts were screened. Nine RCTs were included in the final synthesis. The effect estimate used was weighted average of mean difference (WMD). The results of the meta-analyses showed the treatment was effective in reducing HbA1c in six studies (WMD = 0.56 [0.36–0.75] p < 0.01) and CRP in three studies (WMD = 1.89 [1.70–2.08] p < 0.01). The meta-analyses showed no heterogeneity ($I^2 = 0\%$). Standard treatment of periodontitis by SRP significantly improved glycaemic control and reduced systemic inflammation in persons with type 2 diabetes.

Type 1 diabetes

Type 1 diabetes is insulin-dependent diabetes. It mainly affects young persons. It is believed to be due to immunologic, genetic, and/or environmental causes. Dicembrini, Serni, Monami, Caliri et al. reported in their SR a prevalence of PD of 18.5% (varied from 8.0% to 37.1%) in type 1 diabetes

(23). The OR for PD in type 1 diabetes versus the general population was 2.51 (1.32–4.76, p = 0.005) in comparison to the general population without type 1 diabetes. PD measured by clinical attachment level was more severe in persons with type 1 diabetes but less severe when the patient had good hyperglycaemic control. Ismail, McGrath, and You studied the literature on the oral health of persons with type 1 diabetes (24). In all, 37 studies were included. The authors found some variation between the studies with regard to caries. Most studies reported greater plaque level and more gingivitis. In the cohort studies, no marked differences between children with type 1 diabetes and healthy children with regard to periodontal parameters were reported. Jensen, Allen, Bednarz, Couper et al. conducted a systematic literature search and included 23 studies to assess PD differences in type 1 diabetes children and adolescents versus healthy controls (25). From these studies, the authors reported that children with type 1 diabetes had higher mean values of PI, GI, pocket depth, BOP, and CAL.

Gestational diabetes

For more information on this subject, see Chapter 13 (*Pregnancy and Preterm Birth*). First-time onset of diabetes in pregnancy is termed gestational diabetes mellitus (GDM). This condition has serious complications for the mother and the foetus. Although the aetiology is not well understood, glucose intolerance is an underlying factor. Because periodontitis has implications for the immune system, a possible association has been investigated in several studies. Elevated heterogeneity indicates the need for prospective studies with more homogenous criteria for the diagnoses of periodontitis and diabetes.

Diabetes and root canal treatment

Diabetes is a contributing factor in root canal treatment and need to be taken into account in the treatment of patients with diabetes. Nagendrababu, Segura-Egea, Fouad, Pulikkotil et al. conducted an umbrella review of four SRs on this issue (27). The authors discussed several factors that may explain the results of the included SRs, referring to the described bidirectional relationship between diabetes and periodontitis. Both conditions are related to inflammatory and immunological factors. The primary outcome was the prevalence of persistent apical periodontitis associated with root fillings, which indicates that the endodontic treatment has not succeeded in removing the infection. The authors defined several secondary outcomes: extraction after endodontic treatment, rate of healing assessed by X-rays posttreatment, signs and symptoms after endodontic treatment, survival of teeth, persistent apical periodontitis independent of marginal periodontitis, and level of glycaemia of the patient related to the periapical infection and posttreatment. The results were as follows: The OR of diabetes versus nondiabetes and the prevalence of radiolucent periapical lesions in root filled teeth was 1.44 (1.11–1.80). The risk of diabetes and extracted teeth in relation to root canal treatment was an OR of 2.44 (1.5–3.88). These results show the complications and consequences of root canal treatment in diabetes. This is an important consideration when treating patients with diabetes, and it emphasizes the importance of prophylactic treatment to prevent the need for root canal treatment.

Concluding remarks

There are many studies that confirm the bidirectional relationship of diabetes and periodontitis. There is some heterogeneity between the studies most likely due to differences in recording PD status, type 2 diabetes risk level, and study design. The bidirectional relationship is, to a certain degree, related to both diseases having an important inflammatory component. This relationship is not confirmed in type 1 diabetes. PD in patients with type 1 diabetes has been studied, and results vary. However, patients with type 1 diabetes appear to be at increased risk of more periodontal symptoms than controls. There is conflicting evidence regarding caries.

References

1. Tsalamandris, S, Antonopoulos, AS, Oikonomou, E, Papamikroulis, G-A, Vogiatzi, G, Papaioannou, S, Deftereos, S, and Tousoulis, D. 2019. "The Role of Inflammation in Diabetes: Current Concepts and Future Perspectives." *European Cardiology Review*, No. 14 (1): 50–59. https://dx.doi.org/10.15420/ecr.2018.33.1

2. Chinnasamy, A, and Moodie, M. "Prevalence of Undiagnosed Diabetes and Prediabetes in the Dental Setting: A Systematic Review and Meta-Analysis." *International Journal of Dentistry*, No. 2020: 2964020. https://doi.org/10.1155/2020/2964020

3. Mauri-Obradors, E, Estrugo-Devesa, A, Jané-Salas, E, Viñas, M, and López-López, J. 2017. "Oral Manifestations of Diabetes Mellitus. A Systematic Review." *Medicina Oral, Patologia Oral, Cirugia Bucal*, No. 22 (5): e586–e594. https://doi.org/10.4317/medoral.21655

4.   Liu, LS, Gkranias, N, Farias, B, Spratt, D, and Donos, N. 2018.
     "Differences in the Subgingival Microbial Population of Chronic
     Periodontitis in Subjects with and without Type 2 Diabetes
     Mellitus—a Systematic Review." *Clinical Oral Investigations*, No.
     22(8): 2743–2762. https://doi.org/10.1007/s00784-018-2660-2
5.   Chapple, Iain LC, Genco, Robert, and Working Group 2 of the Joint
     EFP/AAP Workshop. 2013. "Diabetes and Periodontal Diseases:
     Consensus Report of the Joint EFP/AAP Workshop on Periodontitis
     and Systemic Diseases." *Journal of Periodontology*, No. 84 (4
     Suppl): S106–S112. https://doi.org/10.1902/jop.2013.1340011
6.   Graziani, F, Gennai, S, Solini, A, and Petrini, M. 2018. "A Systematic
     Review and Meta-analysis of Epidemiologic Observational Evidence
     on the Effect of Periodontitis on Diabetes: An Update of the EFP-
     AAP Review." *Journal of Clinical Periodontology*, No. 45(2): 167–
     187.
7.   Nascimento, GG, Leite, FRM, Vestergaard, P, Scheutz, F, and
     López, R. 2018. "Does Diabetes Increase the Risk of Periodontitis?
     A Systematic Review and Meta-regression Analysis of Longitudinal
     Prospective Studies." *Acta Diabetologica*, No. 55 (7): 653–667.
     https://doi.org/10.1007/s00592-018-1120-4
8.   Ryan, ME, Carnu, O, and Kamer, A. 2003. "The Influence of
     Diabetes on the Periodontal Tissues." *Journal of the American
     Dental Association*, No. 134 34S–40S.
     https://doi.org/10.14219/jada.archive.2003.0370
9.   Wu, CZ, Yuan, YH, Liu, HH, Li, SS, Zhang, BW, Chen, W, An, ZJ,
     Chen, SY, Wu, YZ, Han, B, Li, CJ, and Li, LJ. 2020. "Epidemiologic
     Relationship between Periodontitis and Type 2 Diabetes Mellitus."
     BMC Oral Health, 20 (1): 204. https://doi.org/10.1186/s12903-020-
     01180-w
10. Ziukaite, L, Slot, DE, and Van der Weijden, FA. 2018. "Prevalence
     of Diabetes Mellitus in People Clinically Diagnosed with
     Periodontitis: A Systematic Review and Meta-analysis of Epidemiologic
     Studies." *Journal of Clinical Periodontology*, No. 45 (6): 650–662.
     https://doi.org/10.1111/jcpe.12839
11. Borgnakke, WS, Ylöstalo, PV, Taylor, GW, and Genco, RJ. 2013.
     "Effect of Periodontal Disease on Diabetes: Systematic Review of
     Epidemiologic Observational Evidence." *Journal of Periodontology*,
     No. 84 (4 Suppl): S135–S152.
     https://doi.org/10.1902/jop.2013.1340013
12. Håheim, Lise L, Rønningen, KS, Enersen, M, and Olsen, I. 2017.
     "The Predictive Role of Tooth Extractions, Oral Infections, and hs-

C-reactive Protein for Mortality in Individuals with and without Diabetes: A Prospective Cohort Study of a 12 1/2-Year Follow-Up." *Journal of Diabetes Research*, No. 2017: 9590740. https://doi.org/10.1155/2017/9590740

13.   Simpson, TC, Weldon, JC, Worthington, HV, Needleman, I, Wild, SH, Moles, DR, Stevenson, B, Furness, S, and Iheozor-Ejiofor, Z. 2015. "Treatment of Periodontal Disease for Glycaemic Control in People with Diabetes Mellitus." *Cochrane Database of Systematic Reviews*, No. 2015 (11): CD004714. https://doi.org/10.1002/14651858.CD004714.pub3

14.   Santos, CM, Lira-Junior, R, Fischer, RG, Santos, AP, and Oliveira, BH. 2015. "Systemic Antibiotics in Periodontal Treatment of Diabetic Patients: A Systematic Review." *PLoS One*, No. 10 (12): e0145262. https://doi.org/10.1371/journal.pone.0145262

15.   Mauri-Obradors, E, Jané-Salas, E, Sabater-Recolons Mdel, M, Viñas, M, and López-López, J. 2015. "Effect of Nonsurgical Periodontal Treatment on Glycosylated Hemoglobin in Diabetic Patients: A Systematic Review." *Odontology*, No. 103 (3): 301–313. https://doi.org/10.1007/s10266-014-0165-2

16.   Botero, JE, Rodríguez, C, and Agudelo-Suarez, AA. 2016. "Periodontal Treatment and Glycaemic Control in Patients with Diabetes and Periodontitis: An Umbrella Review." *Australian Dental Journal*, No. 61 (2): 134–148. https://doi.org/10.1111/adj.12413

17.   Pérez-Losada, FL, Jané-Salas, E, Sabater-Recolons, MM, Estrugo-Devesa, A, Segura-Egea, JJ, and López-López, J. 2016. "Correlation between Periodontal Disease Management and Metabolic Control of Type 2 Diabetes Mellitus. A Systematic Literature Review." *Medicina Oral, Patologia Oral, Cirugia Bucal*, No. 21 (4): e440–e446. https://doi.org/10.4317/medoral.21048

18.   Baeza Hasuike, A, Iguchi, S, Suzuki, D, Kawano, E, and Sato, S. 2017. "Systematic Review and Assessment of Systematic Reviews Examining the Effect of Periodontal Treatment on Glycemic Control in Patients with Diabetes." *Medicina Oral, Patologia Oral, Cirugia Bucal*, No. 22 (2): e167–e176. https://doi.org/10.4317/medoral.21555

19.   Abduljabbar, T, Javed, F, Shah, A, Samer, MS, Vohra, F, and Akram, Z. 2017. "Role of Lasers as an Adjunct to Scaling and Root Planing in Patients with Type 2 Diabetes Mellitus: A Systematic Review." Lasers Med Sci, No. 32 (2): 449–459. https://doi.org/10.1007/s10103-016-2086-5

20.   Cao, R, Li, Q, Wu, Q, Yao, M, Chen, Y, and Zhou, H. 2019. "Effect of Non-surgical Periodontal Therapy on Glycemic Control of Type 2 Diabetes Mellitus: A Systematic Review and Bayesian Network Meta-analysis." *BMC Oral Health*, No. 19 (1): 176. https://doi.org/10.1186/s12903-019-0829-y

21.   Yap, KCH, and Pulikkotil, SJ. 2019. "Systemic Doxycycline as an Adjunct to Scaling and Root Planing in Diabetic Patients with Periodontitis: A Systematic Review and Meta-analysis." *BMC Oral Health*, No. 19 (1): 209. https://doi.org/10.1186/s12903-019-0873-7

22.   Morales, A, Cisterna, C, Cavalla, F, Jara, G, Isamitt, Y, Pino, P, and Gamonal, J. 2020. "Effect of Periodontal Treatment in Patients with Periodontitis and Diabetes: Systematic Review and Meta-analysis." *Journal of Applied Oral Science*, No. 28: e20190248. https://doi.org/10.1590/1678-7757-2019-0248

23.   Dicembrini, I, Serni, L, Monami, M, Caliri, M, Barbato, L, Cairo, F, and Mannucci, E. 2020. "Type 1 Diabetes and Periodontitis: Prevalence and Periodontal Destruction—a Systematic Review." *Acta Diabetologica*, No. 57 (12): 1405–1412. https://doi.org/10.1007/s00592-020-01531-7

24.   Ismail, AF, McGrath, CP, and You, CK. 2015. "Oral Health of Children with Type 1 Diabetes Mellitus: A Systematic Review." *Diabetes Research and Clinical Practice*, No. 108 (3): 369–381. https://doi.org/10.1016/j.diabres.2015.03.003

25.   Jensen, E, Allen, G, Bednarz, J, Couper J, and Peña, A. 2020. "Periodontal Risk Markers in Children and Adolescents with Type 1 Diabetes: A Systematic Review and Meta-analysis." *Diabetes/Metabolism Research and Reviews*, No. 18: e3368. https://doi.org/10.1002/dmrr.3368

26.   Abariga, SA, and Whitcomb, BW. 2016. "Periodontitis and Gestational Diabetes Mellitus: A Systematic Review and Meta-analysis of Observational Studies." *BMC Pregnancy Childbirth*, No. 16 (1): 344. https://doi.org/10.1186/s12884-016-1145-z

27.   Nagendrababu, V, Segura-Egea, JJ, Fouad, AF, Pulikkotil, SJ, and Dummer, PMH. 2020. "Association between Diabetes and the Outcome of Root Canal Treatment in Adults: An Umbrella Review." *International Journal of Endocrinology*. 53 (4): 455-466. https://doi.org/10.1111/iej.13253

Chapter 10

Lung diseases

Microbes are transported to the upper and lower respiratory airways by inhalation or mucous transport. A great number of different virulent organisms cause disease in the airways. Bacterial infections can be acute or can take a chronic course, some requiring antibiotic treatment. Aspiration of oral bacteria from oral infection sites, can cause lung abscess. If antibiotic does not remove the infection, surgery may be required. Viral infections, such as the yearly influenza, can be prevented by vaccination. Although the influenza virus mutates every year, the vaccine is adjusted to respond to the new mutated virus. In December 2019, a new virus was discovered – the COVID-19 virus, a SARS virus causing a pandemic for which there was no a vaccine. The pandemic continued into 2020 and 2021 and has caused a great number of deaths worldwide. Vaccines have been developed, and they will curb the pandemic when a sufficient number of persons has been vaccinated. However, mutations of the virus spread around the world. During the COVID-19 pandemic, the young ones have been spared in contrast to the fragile elderly. The human body has defence mechanisms, such as cilia lining the throat. The minute and numerous filaments continuously move shifting mucous and debris up and out of the throat – nature's protection of the airways. As expected, cilia filaments are most efficient amongst the young and less so through life due to the influence of smoking, alcohol, and possibly different kinds of food, drink, and medication (1).

This chapter will explore the evidence for oral infections being associated with lung diseases. Documentation is available for COVID-19, pneumonia, asthma, cystic fibrosis (CF), and chronic obstructive lung disease. Cancer of the lung is described in Chapter 11 (Cancer).

COVID-19

Since the COVID-19 pandemic started fully in early 2020, research has been (and continues to be) carried out extensively to understand all the elements of the pandemic and disease development. The virus is called SARS-CoV-

2, and it belongs to the Corona family of viruses, which are known to cause respiratory infections leading to light colds or a more serious disease of the lungs and may have a fatal outcome. Presenting symptoms may be one or more of these: Fever or chills, cough, shortness of breath or difficulty breathing, fatigue, muscle or body ache, headache, new loss of taste or smell, sore throat, congestion or runny nose, nausea or vomiting, and/or diarrhea. https://www.cdc.gov/coronavirus/2019-ncov/symptoms-testing/symptoms.html

Regarding oral health in COVID-19 patients, Marouf, Cai, Said, Daas et al. provided some early and interesting observations (2). In a study of 568 patients with COVID-19, the authors observed that patients with periodontitis were 3.5 times more likely to be admitted for intensive care treatment (OR = 3.54, 95% CI 1.39–9.05), 4.6 times more likely to need ventilator treatment (OR = 4.57, 95% CI 1.19–17.4), and 8.8 times more likely to die (OR = 8.81, 95% CI 1.00–77.7) than patients without PD. These results may indicate that the immune system of patients with periodontitis is already, in a sense, overloaded and struggles to cope with the additional COVID-19 infection. It is also speculated that the presence of periodontitis makes the coronavirus more aggressive. The patients in the study with periodontitis had higher levels of inflammatory markers in their blood than patients without periodontitis. Undoubtedly, more research results on COVID-19 will be available in the future.

Pneumonia

Intervention studies studying the effect of removing a risk factor are important in exploring disease causes. The following results illustrate this point. The risk of postoperative pneumonia after cardiac surgery increases the burden of disease for patients. Bardia, Blitz, Dai, Hersey et al. conducted an SR of interventions by giving preoperative chlorhexidine (CHX) mouth rinse, which lowers the bacterial burden in the mouth, to patients with cardiac conditions prior to surgery (3). Eligible literature published until 2017 were included. Five studies (N = 2,284 patients) were included, and 1,125 patients received CHX gluconate as a preoperative mouth rinse (3). The risk of postoperative pneumonia was reduced significantly in this group compared to those who did not receive a mouth rinse (RR = 0.52, 95% CI 0.39–0.70, p < 0.001). No adverse effects from CHX gluconate were reported.

In a Cochrane report, oral hygiene measures such as using a mouth rinse, gel, or swab; tooth brushing; or a combination, together with suction of secretions, were assessed for reduction in ventilator-associated pneumonia (VAP) in patients receiving mechanical ventilation for at least 48 hours (4). In all, 40 RCTs (N = 5,675 participants were included). The studies were divided into five categories of comparisons of oral care: 1) CHX mouth rinse or gel versus placebo/usual care; CHX mouth rinse versus other oral care agents, 2) tooth brushing (± antiseptics) versus no tooth brushing (± antiseptics), 3) powered versus manual tooth brushing, and 4) comparisons of other oral care agents used versus placebo/usual care or 5) head-to-head comparisons between other oral care agents. The results showed no differences for mortality, duration of ventilation, or duration of intensive care unit (ICU) stay. According to five RCTs (n = 910 participants), tooth brushing (+/- antiseptics) may reduce VAP compared to without (RR = 0.61, 95% CI 0.41–0.91, p = 0.01, I^2 = 40%). According to three RCTs, (n = 749 participants), tooth brushing may also reduce ICU stay (WMD -1.89 days, 95% CI -3.52 days – 0.27 days, p = 0.02, I^2 = 0%). The authors concluded that using CHX mouthwash or gel as part of oral hygiene care is beneficial and may reduce VAP in critically ill patients.

Sjögren, Wårdh, Zimmerman, Almståhl et al. studied oral health care in hospitals and nursing homes, comparing care given by dental personnel or general oral care by nursing staff (5). In an SR, the researchers studied the outcome of mortality from healthcare-associated pneumonia in the elderly in hospitals or nursing homes. A meta-analysis was performed for five RCTs, and the dental personnel reduced the risk of mortality (RR = 0.43, 95% CI 0.25–0.76, p = 0.003), whereas oral care interventions given by nursing personnel did not.

Increased risk for nosocomial pneumonia in patients in the ICU by periodontitis was investigated by Jerônimo, Abreu, Cunha, and Esteves Lima (6). They conducted an SR and included 5 case-control studies out of the identified 560 studies. There was a significant association between periodontitis and nosocomial pneumonia in the meta-analysis (OR = 2.55, 95% CI 1.68–3.86, I^2 = 0%). The result showed that patients with periodontitis treated in the ICU were at a higher risk of nosocomial pneumonia than patients without periodontitis.

Another SR was conducted to explore the efficacy of tooth brushing in reducing the risk of VAP (7). Removal of the dental biofilm, plaque, was considered important to prevent VAP. The literature search identified 215 articles, of which 12 were included. They found that different strategies of tooth brushing with or without CHX had been studied, but the pooled estimate was nonsignificant.

Gomes-Filho, Cruz, Trindade, Passos-Soares et al. conducted an SR of studies regarding the association of periodontitis and the following diseases: pneumonia, asthma, and chronic obstructive pulmonary disease (COPD) (8). In all, 10 studies (N = 3,234 participants) were included in the meta-analyses for the three outcomes. For pneumonia, adjusted OR was 3.21 (95% CI 1.997–5.17, $I^2 = 0\%$).

Asthma

In an SR, Gomes-Filho, Cruz, Trindade, Passos-Soares et al. found that periodontitis was associated with asthma (adjusted OR = 3.54, 95% CI 2.47–5.07, $I^2 = 0\%$) (8). Ferreira, Ferreira, Castro, Magno et al. conducted an SR to study the association between PD and asthma in adults using results of observational studies (9). Persons with asthma were compared with persons without asthma. In all, 3,395 studies were identified and reviewed. Eleven studies were included in the SR, and six were used for quantitative analyses. The meta-analyses were performed according to the following clinical parameters: plaque index (PI), gingival index (GI), bleeding on probing (BOP), papillary bleeding index, calculus index, and clinical attachment loss (CAL). The results for the calculus index was $p < 0.00001$ and $I^2 = 0\%$; for the papillary bleeding index, $p < 0.00001$ and $I^2 = 0\%$; and for the CAL, $p = 0.03$ and $I^2 = 98\%$, all significantly higher in persons with asthmatic disease than in persons without asthma. Nonsignificant associations were found for BOP, GI, and PI. The results indicate that persons with asthma have more periodontitis and gingivitis than persons without asthma.

Similarly, Moraschini, Calasans-Maia, and Calasans-Maia wrote an SR on the association of PD and asthma (10). They searched for studies of different designs, including prospective and retrospective cohort studies, case-controls, and randomized clinical trials, published between 1979 and 2017. They authors found significant associations for clinical evidence of gingivitis as gingival bleeding, PI, and GI for participants with asthma ($p < 0.001$).

Cystic fibrosis

CF is a lung disorder, and more information can be found on the following website or other websites: https://www.medicalnewstoday.com/articles/147960. 'Cystic fibrosis is a hereditary disease that affects the lungs and digestive system. The body produces thick and sticky mucus that can clog the lungs and obstruct the pancreas. Cystic fibrosis (CF) can be life-threatening'.

In CF, the lung condition presents with thick and sticky mucus. Persons with CF need close follow-up and antibiotic treatment more often for lung infections. Coffey, O'Leary, Burke, Roberts et al. (2020) conducted an SR of studies to assess how the periodontal condition was for persons with CF (11), evaluating if there was an added risk due to poor oral health. The authors included 13 studies in a qualitative review. Most of the studies indicated that cases with CF had better oral hygiene than controls but did have more calculus. In one study involving children, they found more gingivitis among the cases, and in another, the cases had more BOP. One study included adults only, five studies included persons over 18 years, and most of the studies included children only. In 2019, Pawlaczyk-Kamieńska, Borysewicz-Lewicka, Śniatała, Batura-Gabryel et al. focussed their SR on dental disease and PD (12). These two reviews overlap in many respects.

Chronic obstructive pulmonary disease

Gomes-Filho, Cruz, Trindade, Passos-Soares et al. conducted an SR of studies on the association of periodontitis with pneumonia, asthma, and chronic obstructive pulmonary disease (COPD) (8). The results for COPD was as follows: adjusted OR = 1.78 (95% CI 1.04–3.05) and $I^2 = 38\%$.

Concluding remarks

Oral bacteria do get aspirated into the bronchi and lungs. This is more serious for some patient groups than others. The study results presented in this chapter indicate that persons with asthma have poorer oral health than persons with CF. Intervention studies involving persons on ventilators have been carried out, and oral hygiene measures have been shown to be effective in preventing nosocomial pneumonia in these seriously ill patients.

References

1.   Håheim, Lise L. 2020. "Epithelial Cilia Is the First Line of Defence against Coronavirus; Addressing the Observed Age-Gradient in the COVID-19 Infection." *Medical Hypotheses*. 143: oct 2020. https://doi.org/10.1016/j.mehy.2020.110064

2.   Marouf, N, Cai, W, Said, KN, Daas, H, Diab, H, Chinta, BR, Hssain, Ali A, Nicolau, B, Sanz, M, and Tamimi, F. 2021. "Association

between Periodontitis and Severity of COVID-19 Infection: A Case-Control Study." *Journal of Clinical Periodontology*. 48 (4):483-491. https://doi.org/10.1111/jcpe.13435

3.   Bardia, A, Blitz, D, Dai, F, Hersey, D, Jinadasa, S, Tickoo, M, and Schonberger, RB. 2019. "Preoperative Chlorhexidine Mouthwash to Reduce Pneumonia after Cardiac Surgery: A Systematic Review and Meta-analysis." *Journal of Thoracic and Cardiovascular Surgery*, No. 158: 1094–1100.

4.   Zhao, T, Wu, X, Zhang, Q, Li, C, Worthington, HV, and Hua, F. 2020. "Oral Hygiene Care for Critically Ill Patients to Prevent Ventilator-Associated Pneumonia." *Cochrane Database of Systematic Reviews*, No. 12: CD008367.

5.   Sjögren, P, Wårdh, I, Zimmerman, M, Almståhl, A, and Wikström, M. 2016. "Oral Care and Mortality in Older Adults with Pneumonia in Hospitals or Nursing Homes: Systematic Review and Meta-analysis." *Journal of the American Geriatrics Society*, No. 64: 2109–2115.

6.   Jerônimo, LS, Abreu, LG, Cunha, FA, and Esteves Lima, RP. 2020. "Association between Periodontitis and Nosocomial Pneumonia: A Systematic Review and Meta-analysis of Observational Studies." *Oral Health and Preventive Dentistry*, No. 18: 11–17.

7.   de Camargo, L, da Silva, SN, and Chambrone, L. 2019. "Efficacy of Toothbrushing Procedures Performed in Intensive Care Units in Reducing the Risk of Ventilator-Associated Pneumonia: A Systematic Review." *Journal of Periodontal Research*, No. 54: 601–611.

8.   Gomes-Filho, IS, Cruz, SSD, Trindade, SC, Passos-Soares, JS, Carvalho-Filho, PC, Figueiredo, ACMG, Lyrio, AO, Hintz, AM, Pereira, MG, and Scannapieco, F. 2020. "Periodontitis and Respiratory Diseases: A Systematic Review with Meta-analysis." *Oral Diseases*, No. 26: 439–446.

9.   Ferreira, MKM, Ferreira, RO, Castro, MML, Magno, MB, Almeida, APCPSC, Fagundes, NCF, Maia, LC, and Lima, RR. 2019. "Is There an Association between Asthma and Periodontal Disease among Adults? Systematic Review and Meta-analysis." *Life Sciences*, No. 223: 74–87.

10.   Moraschini, V, Calasans-Maia, JA, and Calasans-Maia, MD. 2018. "Association between Asthma and Periodontal Disease: A Systematic Review and Meta-analysis." *Journal of Periodontology*, No. 89: 440–455.

11. Coffey, N, O'Leary, F, Burke, F, Roberts, A, and Hayes, M. 2020. "Periodontal and Oral Health Status of People with Cystic Fibrosis: A Systematic Review." *Journal of Dentistry*, No. 103: 103509.
12. Pawlaczyk-Kamieńska, T, Borysewicz-Lewicka, M, Śniatała, R, Batura-Gabryel, H, and Cofta, S. 2019. "Dental and Periodontal Manifestations in Patients with Cystic Fibrosis – a Systematic Review." *Journal of Cystic Fibrosis*, No. 18: 762–771.

CHAPTER 11

CANCER

Oral cancer has been studied for a long time, but how the normal oral microbiota has been involved in the pathophysiology is less certain, nor is the pathophysiology of oral disease to cancers originating distant to the oral cavity fully understood. So far, the link most studied is the pathology related to immunology and the infection route.

The most common oral infections are gingivitis, periodontitis, and caries; all start with bacteria forming a biofilm on the tooth and gingival surfaces. The infections proceed to destroy soft and hard tissues of the jaws due to anaerobic bacteria; hence, tooth extraction is a measure of this disease. Bacteria find nutrients in saliva and the food we eat. The biofilm, also termed plaque, can calcify after adherence to the tooth surface. The progress of these diseases is well understood, but from there to the initiation of cancer is a more complex pathology. This does not only apply to the risk of oral cancers but also applies to cancers of distant sites, making oral infections and their "components" possible risk factors unless they are prevented and/or treated. Several risk assessments have been performed in different studies, depending on the scientific hypotheses, available data, and the opportunity to design and carry out new research mainly from laboratory studies, health surveys, clinical examinations, cohort studies, case-control studies, and/or registry data.

In the following, results will be presented mainly from SRs of scientific literature with meta-analyses including several studies but also results from single studies. The included study designs are prospective cohort, case-control, nested case control, and case-cohort. There is a limited overlap of some studies regarding the specific cancer diagnoses, as these have been used in more than one SR. Confounding factors are always an issue. Age and smoking, in addition to socioeconomic status, are important in both periodontitis and cancer. Education is a proxy for knowledge on infection prevention, and frequency of visits to the dentist reflects treatment and prophylaxis against the common oral infections and the availability of dental services and cost.

This chapter starts with the risk posed by specific oral pathogens, following self-reported PD found to be associated with the overall risk of cancer, and continues with specific cancer diagnoses. Total cancer reflects different gender-specific cancer diagnoses, and cancer-specific results are an advantage. More research is needed to identify serum markers that may help in developing tests for screening and early diagnosis and possibly be used in following the prognosis and management of cancers.

Oral pathogens in cancer

Periodontal bacteria are the major pathogens in the oral cavity and the main cause of adult chronic periodontitis, but their association with incidence and prognosis in cancer is controversial. The aim of the study by Xiao, Zhang, Peng, Wang et al. (2020) was to evaluate the effect of periodontal bacterial infection on the incidence and prognosis of cancer (1). Their research included 39 studies presented in 18 articles comprising 7,184 participants. The studies came from different countries: 16 came from Asia, 19 from North America, and 3 from Europe. The authors found results indicating that periodontal bacterial infection increases the incidence of cancer (OR = 1.25, 95% CI 1.03–1.52, I^2 = 70%) and is associated with poor overall survival (HR = 1.75, 95% CI 1.40–2.20), disease-free survival (HR = 2.18, 95% CI 1.24–3.84), and cancer-specific survival (HR = 1.85, 95% CI 1.44–2.39). The samples were taken from blood, saliva, mouthwash, tissues, or serum, and detection was by 16S rRNA gene sequencing, quantitative PCR, ELISA, or droplet digital PCR. Subgroup analysis indicated that cancer risk was associated with *Porphyromonas gingivalis* (Pg) infection (OR = 2.16, 95% CI 1.34–3.47) (10 studies) and *Prevotella intermedia* (Pi) infection (OR = 1.28, 95% CI 1.01–1.63) (2 studies) but not *Tannerella forsythia* (Tf) (OR = 1.06, 95% CI 0.8–1.41) (5 studies), *Treponema denticola* (Td) (OR = 1.30, 95% CI 0.99–1.72) (3 studies), *Aggregatibacter actinomycetemcomitans* (Aa) (OR = 1.00, 95% CI 0.48–2.08) (3 studies) or *Fusobacterium nucleatum* (Fn) infections (OR = 0.61, 95% CI 0.32–1.16) (15 studies). The authors concluded that the meta-analysis revealed that periodontal bacterial infection increases the incidence of cancer and predicts poor prognosis for cancer development.

In 2016, Sayehmiri, Sayehmiri, Asadollahi, Soroush et al., in their meta-analysis, explored studies that had evaluated the prevalence rate of the bacterium Pg in patients with gingival cancer (2). From eight studies (2000–2013), the authors noticed a nonsignificant increased risk for cancer (OR= 1.36, 95% CI 0.47–3.97, I^2 = 81.5%). Pg prevalence in four case-control studies was 40.7% (95% CI 19.3–62.1), which indicates the prevalence of chronic periodontitis in cancer patients. Pg is one of the red complex bacteria in chronic periodontitis and, as such, is interesting to study in cancer pathology. The authors listed several potentially carcinogenic properties of Pg.

In 2017, Bracci wrote a review of epidemiologic studies to evaluate PD, different oral microbiome parameters, and the risk of pancreatic cancer (3). The studies showed risk estimates ranging from 1.5 to 2.0, with an overall RR of 1.74. Antibodies to oral commensal bacteria were analysed from prediagnostic blood samples to estimate any predictive effect. In conclusion, Bracci pointed to the complexity of possible pathology by assessing the oral microbiome, periodontitis, and other risk factors – realizing the involvement of the immune and inflammatory processes, which needs to be studied further.

Self-assessed or self-reported periodontitis

Michaud, Fu, Shi, and Chung (2017) wrote an SR of cohort and case-control studies and conducted a meta-analysis of the risk estimates (4). From 11 former reviews, the authors identified 52 studies, and through a PubMed search for the period 2011 to 2016, they identified 217 studies and 18 relevant abstracts. Studies were excluded for the following reasons: they were duplicates, no exposure or outcome was of interest, the study design was not relevant, no adjustment of the results for confounders, or not all participants had established periodontitis. Of the finally selected 46 studies, the authors found risk estimates, enabling them to perform separate meta-analyses for total cancer and for lung, head and neck, pancreas, stomach and oesophagus, breast, and colorectal cancers. The authors' requirements for studies to be included in the meta-analyses were the risk of having PD or tooth numbers as a surrogate for PD and that the study estimates had been adjusted for smoking. In their paper, the authors presented figures of two meta-analyses, one on results of lung cancer and the other on cancer of the pancreas (see results in the separate cancer specific paragraphs).

Corbella, Veronesi, Galimberti, Weinstein et al. (2018) adopted another approach for studying periodontitis and the development of cancer. They reviewed 490 papers, and after a systematic assessment, 10 papers from 6 studies (prospective cohorts and case-control studies) were included in their meta-analyses (5). Corbella, Veronesi, Galimberti, Weinstein et al. assessed the cancer risk by HRs from Cox proportional hazard regression analyses. All 10 papers were included in the qualitative synthesis and 8 in the quantitative synthesis; the eight papers covered six studies. Separate analyses were performed for any cancer, including cancers of the digestive tract, pancreatic, prostate, breast, corpus uteri, and lungs; haematological and oesophagus/oropharyngeal combined cancers; and non-Hodgkin cancers, and these results are included in the specific cancer paragraphs below (Table 1).

Table 1. Overview of included studies in the systematic review on cancer and periodontitis by Corbella, Veronesi, Galimberti, Weinstein et al. (5)

First author, year of publication, location, data source (reference no.)	Number of participants		Oral risk factors	Confounder adjusted	Cancer diagnosis
	Men	Women			
Arora (2010), Sweden, Swedish Twin Registry (8)	6,900	8,433	Self-assessed in 1963. Forty-one years of follow-up	Gender, age, education, employment, number of siblings, smoking status, smoking status of partner, alcohol status, diabetes, and body mass index	Any cancer Digestive tract Colorectal Pancreas Stomach Bladder Prostate Breast Corpus uteri Lungs
Eliot (2013), US, nine medical facilities in the Boston area (9)	797	283	Self-assessed follow-up	Age, gender, race, smoking, alcohol status, education, and annual household income	Oral Pharynx Larynx

Mai (2014), US, Women's Health Initiative Observational Study (7)		93,676	Self-assessed follow-up	Age, smoking, education, race, BMI, alcohol, hormone use, dental visits, physical activity, region of residence, and aspirin use	Lungs Breast
Michaud (2007, 2008, 2016), US, Male Health Professionals Study (7)	51,329		Self-assessed follow-up	Main factors: Age, race, BMI, diabetes, profession, smoking, residence area, height, NSAID use, cholecystectomy, multivitamin use, teeth numbers, diet elements, and alcohol	2007 – Pancreas 2008 – Any cancer 2016 – Any cancer
Momen-Harevi (2017), US, Nurse's Health Study (13)		77,443	Self-assessed follow-up	Age, race, smoking, family history of colorectal cancer, diabetes, diet elements, and alcohol	Colorectal
Mazul (2017) US, Carolina Head and Neck Cancer Epidemiology Study (14)	841	383	Self-assessed follow-up	Age, race, sex, alcohol use, socioeconomic status (income, insurance and education), and HPV status	Head and neck squamous cell carcinoma

Total cancer

For total cancer, Michaud, Fu, Shi, and Chung found five prospective cohorts that investigated PD, but only three studies had adjusted for the results of smoking (4). They found that total risk ranged from 14% to 20% in the three studies with analyses controlled for smoking, and the association was consistent across the five studies. From two cohort studies among nonsmokers the results were: In HPFS, a study on men, significant increased risk for total cancer was observed of a HR=1.21 (95% CI 1.06–1.39) (6). In a cohort study on women – the Buffalo OsteoPerio Study (15) – no significant association was found. Missing teeth was not found to be associated with total cancer risk. Corbella, Veronesi, Galimberti, Weinstein et al. found a statistically significant association of PD for all cancers (HR = 1.14, 95% CI 1.04–1.24) (5).

Head and neck cancer

Cancer of the lip and oral cavity is the 15th most common cancer in the world, and the third most common in some Asia Pacific countries (https://www.who.int/news-room/fact-sheets/detail/oral-health). Survival, which reflects treatment, has changed over the years. Radiation treatment to head and neck influences dental status, and patients are, as a rule, treated for dental diseases before radiation treatment starts. The treatment effect and survival are also influenced by the cause of the oral cancer. Cancer due to smoking is more difficult to treat due to the different chemical substances in tobacco and tobacco smoke. Oral cancer due to human papilloma virus (HPV), which is on the increase, is easier to treat and has better survival rates.

As for any cancer, survival the longest is important. Farquhar, Divaris, Mazul, Weissler et al. (16) investigated whether oral health/oral hygiene measures have an influence on surviving head and neck cancers. They did a case-control study of participants of the Carolina Head and Neck Cancer Epidemiologic Study. Cases (n – 1,381) and controls (n = 1,396) that were age-, sex-, and race-matched were followed up for mortality for five years. The oral health indicator was frequency of routine dental examinations and tooth brushing. The researchers found that more than 10 routine dental visits in the 10 years preceding the study decreased the mortality risk by 40% (HR = 0.6 [0.4–0.8]). The reduced risk was strongest for cancers of the oral cavity (HR = 0.4, 95% CI 0.2–0.9). Dental visits were also positive for control persons. Frequent dental visits represents a source of detection bias regarding the results on survival. No other health examinations influenced survival. The results indicate that oral health may have an influence on these cancers through bacteriological and/or immunological pathways.

Guntinas-Lichius, Wendt, Kornetzky, Buentzel et al. (2014) presented data form the Thuringian Cancer Registry, Germany, on the epidemiology and treatment outcome for head and neck cancers for the period 1996–2011 (17).

The authors concluded that overall survival did not improve in this period, but incidence increased significantly.

Chang, Lee, Hsiao, Ovidrelle et al. investigated the oral hygiene habits of regular dental visits, frequency of tooth brushing, and use of dental floss with the aim of removing and controlling the oral microbiome (18). The researchers followed 740 patients with head and neck cancer and found that poor oral hygiene was associated with poor overall survival (HR = 1.38, 95% CI: 1.03–1.86). In addition, they found an association with nucleotide polymorphism (TLR4 rs11536889) and with the CG or CC genotype but not the GG genotype. Based on these results the authors suggest that poor oral hygiene may be a prognostic factor for head and neck cancer.

Periodontal infection

Studies on head and neck cancers are heterogeneous, particularly in terms of risk measurement by extractions or missing teeth, different periodontal measures of the degree of periodontal infection, periodontal pocket depth, and bone loss assessed by radiographs (Michaud, Fu, Shi, and Chung 2017) (4). One cohort study showed a nonsignificant relationship between PD and head and neck cancers. A strong relationship was observed (HR = 2.25, 95% CI 1.30–3.90) of PD for oropharyngeal and oesophageal cancers combined among nonsmokers. The authors did not perform a meta-analysis due to this heterogeneity between studies. However, they presented a figure based on seven case-control studies on the predicted linear dose-response relationship between tooth number and oral cancer (OR = 0.3; 95% CI 0.01–0.05) per tooth lost.

Virus

With smoking cessation taking effect, oral squamous cell carcinoma (OSCC) was on the decrease, until an increase was observed. This increase is caused by Human papilloma virus (HPV) as a result of the sexual behaviour of men in particular. HPV is associated with cancer of the cervix in women and is a risk factor for this carcinoma independent of tobacco and alcohol use. Ribeiro, Levi, Pawlita, Koifman et al. (2011) studied HPV prevalence assessed by HPV DNA in head and neck squamous cell carcinomas in two comparable studies, one in Europe and one in Latin America (20). The results of 2,214 cases versus 3,319 controls indicate a prevalence of HPV E7 DNA (3.1% (6/196) among cases), and serum antibodies were observed in these studies. Several HPV types have been identified in the oral mucosa – including subtypes 1, 2, 6, 7, 11, and 13, as reported by Dai, Clifford, lc Calvez, Castellsagué et al. (2004) regarding the relationship between HPV and oral cancer (21).

Leung, Chung, Yuen, Ho et al. (1995) examined the Epstein–Barr virus and salivary duct cancer in 10 cases, 8 cancers of the parotid gland and 2 of the submandibular gland (19). The authors identified Epstein–Barr virus-encoded small RNAs (EBERs) and all specimens were positive.

Bacteriology and immunology

Park, Woo, Lee, Yoon et al. studied antibody levels to Pg, Fn, and IL-6 which were elevated in OSCC (22). Fn had previously been identified as an emerging factor in colon cancer progression. The authors found Pg and IL-6 to be significantly higher in oral cancer cases (n = 62) compared to controls (n = 46). The authors suggested these factors may be used in the estimation of prognosis.

Lung cancer

The major risk factor for lung cancer is smoking, and the recording of smoking pattern must be as accurate as possible in research studies. Michaud, Fu, Shi, and Chung did a systematic review and found the risk posed by PD in five studies ranging between 1.25 and 4.61, and the pooled RR was 1.33 (95% CI 1.19–1.49) (4). Two studies were on both sexes, two on men only, and one on women only. As smoking is associated with PD and lung cancer, subgroup analyses among nonsmokers were done in the HPFS on men (HR = 0.92, 95% CI 0.49–1.71). Moreover, there was no association with lung cancer in the Women's Health Initiative Observational Study. A significantly higher risk was observed for a higher number of missing teeth after adjusting for smoking dose. A case-cohort study reported a positive association between number of teeth and lung cancer risk. Two of the four case-cohort studies showed a modest nonsignificant increase with a higher number of missing teeth, adjusted for smoking. A large case-control study showed a positive association with a high number of missing teeth.

Corbella, Veronesi, Galimberti, Weinstein et al. found three studies with a risk estimate for periodontitis and associated with lung cancer in their meta-analysis to be an HR of 1.24 (1.06–1.45, $I^2 = 0\%$) (5).

Breast cancer

Breast cancer is the most common cancer among women. It is an endocrinal disorder, and the use of the birth prevention pill and reproduction history have been scrutinized in relation to causation. High BMI and physical activity are other factors that have been studied, but risk factor patterns have not been clarified. Regarding breast cancer, tumours are analysed for three receptors – HER2 (a growth-promoting protein on the outside of all breast cells), oestrogen receptor, and progesterone receptors – that will influence the choice of further treatment to improve survival (24).

Michaud, Fu, Shi, and Chung (2017) identified five cohort studies but did not report any significant associations of PD with breast cancer. The risk estimate ranged from 0.94 to 1.32 (4).

Shi, Min, Sun, Zhang et al. conducted a meta-analysis of PD as a predictor of breast cancer based on eight cohort studies (N = 168,111 participants) and found an RR of 1.18 (95% CI 1.11–1.26, I^2 = 17.6%) (25). This is a modest but consistent association. The studies were performed in different European countries.

Corbella, Veronesi, Galimberti, Weinstein et al. assessed the risk of breast cancer by periodontitis to be an HR of 1.11 (95% CI 1.00–1.23) in their meta-analysis (5).

Stomach and oesophageal cancers

As reported earlier, Michaud, Fu, Shi, and Chung (2017) did not report any significant associations (4).

Corbella, Veronesi, Galimberti, Weinstein et al. assessed oesophagus/oropharynx cancer pooled together, and their meta-analysis showed an HR of 2.25 (95% CI 1.30–3.90) (5).

Pancreatic cancer

Increased pancreatic cancer risk was observed in comparing periodontitis with gingivitis (not adjusted for smoking) (OR = 1.2, 95% CI 1.0–2.4) but not for tooth loss in one study (4). Other results were inconsistent, and no meta-analysis was performed. The reason may be study size, no adjustment for smoking in the analyses, differences in study populations, and/or risk measurements performed differently.

More information can be gained from the SR by Maisonneuve Amar, and Lowenfels (2017) (26). They published a review of periodontitis and edentulous or severe teeth loss and risk prediction for pancreatic cancer. From the initial review of 327 references, they selected eight studies. The result of the meta-analyses of six studies (2003–2016) on the risk of periodontitis was an RR of 1.74 (95% CI 1.41–2.15). The risk estimate by edentulous or severe teeth loss from four studies was an RR of 1.54 (95% CI 1.16–2.05). The authors made an interesting comparison of known risk factors for pancreatic cancer and periodontal infection, in addition to tobacco smoking, alcohol consumption, obesity, metabolic syndrome, and allergy (inverse risk).

Diabetes is an associated risk factor for pancreatic cancer, but a direct association with periodontitis is more uncertain. In two studies, Corbella, Veronesi, Galimberti, Weinstein et al. found a risk effect by periodontitis to be an HR of 1.74 (95% CI 1.21–2.52, $I^2 = 0\%$) (5).

Stolzenberg-Solomon, Dodd, Blaser, Virtamo et al. (2003) examined whether tooth loss and/or *Helicobacter pylori* is associated to pancreatic cancer (27). Their hypothesis was tested using data from the Alpha-Tocopherol, Beta-Carotene Cancer Prevention Study cohort in Finland. Edentulous individuals were compared to people with 0–10 teeth missing. Tooth loss was associated with pancreatic cancer (HR = 1.63, 95% CI 1.09–2.46), but *H. pylori* was not.

Oral microbiology

Michaud, Izard, Wilhelm-Benartzi, You et al. (2013) studied plasma antibodies to 25 oral bacteria and pancreatic cancer (28). The work was based on a large multicentre study – the European Prospective Investigation into Cancer and Nutrition study. In a nested case-control study of 405 pancreatic cancer cases and 416 matched controls, the researchers discovered that high levels of Pg resulted in an increased risk of pancreatic cancer (HR = 2.14, 95% CI 1.05–4.36). They also explored the level of antibodies to a cluster of commensal (nonpathogenic) oral bacteria and found an OR of 0.55 (95% CI 0.36–0.83) – indicating high levels of antibodies, compared to low levels, had a 45% lower risk of pancreatic cancer.

Colorectal cancer

The summary estimate of colorectal cancer in four cohorts was an OR of 1.49 (95% CI 0.95–2.29, I^2 = 66.5%) (4). As noted, the risk was nonsignificant. The studies included both sexes or male or female only. The following are included studies on colorectal cancer were Michaud, Liu, Meyer, Giovannucci et al. (6), Arora, Weuve, Fall, Pedersen et al. (8), Mai, LaMonte, Hovey, Freudenheim et al. (15), and Ahn, Segers, and Hayes (29).

Corbella, Veronesi, Galimberti, Weinstein et al. assessed colorectal cancer risk using three studies and found a risk estimate of 0.94 (95% CI 0.79–1.12). The researchers assessed digestive tract cancer and found an HR of 1.34 (95% CI 1.05–1.72) (5). Stomach cancer risk was nonsignificant (HR = 1.03, 95% CI 0.71–1.48).

Bladder cancer

Two studies found bladder cancer risk to be nonsignificant in a meta-analysis (HR = 1.31, 95% CI 0.93–1.84) (5).

Prostate cancer

The only study reporting results of a meta-analysis on prostate cancer was Corbella, Veronesi, Galimberti, Weinstein et al., who found the risk effect by PD to be an HR of 1.25 (95% CI 1.04–1.51, I^2 = 16.0%) in two studies (5).

Corpus uteri cancer

Corbella, Veronesi, Galimberti, Weinstein et al. (2018) found the risk estimate to be an HR of 2.20 (95% CI 1.16–4.18) for corpus uteri cancer (4)

Haematopoietic and lymphatic cancer

Wu, Shi, Li, Shi et al. presented results on the correlation between PD and haematopoietic and lymphatic cancers (30). Their literature search identified 853 papers, and 6 studies were included. Among these were one case-control study from Sweden, one retrospective cohort from China, and four prospective cohorts from the US, all published since 2010. The overall risk estimate of the meta-analysis was an RR of 1.17 (95% CI 1.07–1.27, I^2 = 22.7%). From the subgroup analyses, the researchers found that nonsmokers had an RR of 1.28 (95% CI 1.07–1.54, $I^2 = 0\%$), and the RR for the American population was 1.17 (95% CI 1.0–1.3, $I^2 = 44.8\%$).

Corbella, Veronesi, Galimberti, Weinstein et al. assessed and, in their meta-analysis, calculated HRs of 1.30 (95% CI 1.11–1.53) and 1.30 (95% CI 1.11–1.52) for haematological cancer and non-Hodgkin lymphoma, respectively (5).

Summary of the literature on cancer and oral health

One tends to consider oral infections as one factor causing oral diseases. However, different measures, as outlined, have been used to characterize the oral influence on cancer. Different pathological mechanisms are in play, many of which there is currently insufficient information about. These may be of microbiologic, immunological, genetic, or other causes. What particular factor(s) in the immunologic system is/are important and what characterizes individuals is still mostly uncertain. Studying antibodies to oral bacteria is one track to follow as low levels of antibodies entail the systemic spread of infections. For periodontitis, this may also reflect the differences in individuals' socioeconomic situations. In this chapter, SRs are mainly used, summarizing the results of different studies. A weakness of this approach is the heterogeneity of disease measurements and outcome registration between the studies. This variation results in low risk estimates. If the risk estimate is close to one but significant, it is likely there is an unmeasured risk factor that has not been considered.

Concluding remarks

A classic comment is appropriate here – more research is needed. The different forms of cancer are diverse. Other known risk factors need to be considered regarding the effect of oral infections, especially chronic periodontitis. The results presented indicate some pathological effects by oral microbes and their bacterial products.

References

1.   Xiao, L, Zhang, Q, Peng, Y, Wang, D, and Liu, Y. 2020. "The Effect of Periodontal Bacteria Infection on Incidence and Prognosis of Cancer: A Systematic Review and Meta-analysis." *Medicine (Baltimore)*, No. 99: e19698.
https://doi.org/10.1097/MD.0000000000019698

2. Sayehmiri, F, Sayehmiri, K, Asadollahi, K, Soroush, S, Bogdanovic, L, Azizi Jalilian, F, Emaneini, M, and Taherikalani, M. 2015. "The Prevalence Rate of *Porphyromonas gingivalis* and Its Association with Cancer: A Systematic Review and Meta-analysis." *International Journal of Immunopathology and Pharmacology*, No. 28: 160–167. https://doi.org/10.1177/0394632015586144

3. Bracci, PM. 2017. "Oral Health and the Oral Microbiome in Pancreatic Cancer: An Overview of Epidemiological Studies." *Cancer Journal*, No. 23: 310–314. https://doi.org/10.1097/PPO.0000000000000287

4. Michaud, DS, Fu, X, Shi, J, and Chung, M. 2017. "Periodontal Disease, Tooth Loss, and Cancer Risk." *Epidemiologic Reviews*, No. 39: 49–58. https://doi.org/10.1093/epirev/mxx006

5. Corbella, S, Veronesi, P, Galimberti, V, Weinstein, R, Del Fabbro, M, and Francetti, L. 2018. "Is Periodontitis a Risk Indicator for Cancer? A Meta-analysis." *PLoS One*, No. 13: e0195683. https://doi.org/10.1371/journal.pone.0195683

6. Michaud, DS, Liu, Y, Meyer, M, Giovannucci, E, and Joshipura, K. 2008. "Disease, Tooth Loss and Cancer Risk in a Prospective Study of Male Health Professionals." *Lancet Oncology*, No. 9: 550–558. https://doi.org/10.1016/S1470-2045(08)70106-2

7. Mai, X, LaMonte, MJ, Hovey, KM, Nwizu, N, Freudenheim, JL, Tezal, M, Scannapieco, F, Hyland, A, Andrews, CA, Genco, RJ, and Wactawski-Wende, J. 2014. "History of Periodontal Disease Diagnosis and Lung Cancer Incidence in the Women's Health Initiative Observational Study." *Cancer Causes & Control*, No. 25 (8): 1045–1053.

8. Arora, M, Weuve, J, Fall, K, Pedersen, NL, and Mucci, LA. 2010. "An Exploration of Shared Genetic Risk Factors between Periodontal Disease and Cancers: A Prospective Co-twin Study." *American Journal of Epidemiology*, No. 171(2): 253–259. https://doi.org/10.1093/aje/kwp340

9. Eliot, MN, Michaud, DS, Langevin, SM, McClean, MD, and Kelsey, KT. 2013. "Periodontal Disease and Mouthwash Use Are Risk Factors for Head and Neck Squamous Cell Carcinoma." *Cancer Causes & Control*, No. 24: 1315–1322.

10. Michaud, DS, Joshipura, K, Giovannucci, E, and Joshipura, K. 2007. "A Prospective Study of Periodontal Disease and Pancreatic Cancer in US Male Health Professionals." *Journal of the National Cancer Institute*, No. 99: 171–175.

11.   Michaud, DS, Kelsey, KT, Papathanasiou, E, Genco, CA, and
       Giovannucci, E. 2016. "Periodontal Disease and Risk of All Cancers
       among Male Never Smokers: An Updated Analysis of the Health
       Professionals Follow-Up Study." *Annals of Oncology*, No. 27: 941–
       947. https://doi.org/10.1093/annonc/mdw028
12.   Bertrand, KA, Shingala, J, Evens, A, Birmann, BM, Giovannucci, E,
       and Michaud, DS. 2017. "Periodontal Disease and Risk of Non-
       Hodgkin lymphoma in the Health Professionals Follow-Up Study."
       International Journal of Cancer, No. 140: 1020–1026.
       https://doi.org/10.1002/ijc.30518
13.   Momen-Heravi, F, Babic, A, Tworoger, SS, Zhang, L, Wu, K,
       Smith-Warner, SA, Ogino, S, Chan, AT, Meyerhardt, J,
       Giovannucci, E, Fuchs, C, Cho, E, Michaud, DS, Stampfer, MJ, Yu,
       YH, Kim, D, and Zhang, X. 2017. "Periodontal Disease, Tooth Loss
       and Colorectal Cancer Risk: Results from the Nurses' Health Study."
       International Journal of Cancer, No. 140: 646–652.
       https://doi.org/10.1002/ijc.30486
14.   Mazul, AL, Taylor, JM, Divaris, K, Weissler, MC, Brennan, P,
       Anantharaman, D, Behnoush Abedi-Ardekani, B, Olshan, AF, and
       Zevallos, JP. 2017. "Oral Health and Human Papillomavirus-
       Associated Head and Neck Squamous Cell Carcinoma." *Cancer*, No.
       123: 71–80. https://doi.org/10.1002/cncr.30312
15.   Mai, X, LaMonte, MJ, Hovey, KM, Freudenheim, JL, Andrews, CA,
       Genco, RJ, and Wactawski-Wende, J. 2016. "Periodontal Disease
       Severity and Cancer Risk in Postmenopausal Women: The Buffalo
       OsteoPerio Study." *Cancer Causes & Control*, No. 27: 217–228.
16.   Farquhar, DR, Divaris, K, Mazul, AL, Weissler, MC, Zevallos, JP,
       and Olshan, AF. 2017. "Poor Oral Health Affects Survival in Head
       and Neck Cancer." *Oral Oncology*, No. 73: 111 117.
       https://doi.org/10.1016/j.oraloncology.2017.08.009
17.   Guntinas-Lichius, O, Wendt, TG, Kornetzky, N, Buentzel, J, Esser,
       D, Böger, D, Müller, A, Schultze-Mosgau, S, Schlattmann, P, and
       Schmalenberg, H. 2014. "Trends in Epidemiology and Treatment
       and Outcome for Head and Neck Cancer: A Population-Based Long-
       Term Analysis from 1996 to 2011 of the Thuringian Cancer
       Registry." *Oral Oncology*, No. 50: 1157–1164.
       https://doi.org/10.1016/j.oraloncology.2014.09.015
18.   Chang, CC, Lee, WT, Hsiao, JR, Ovidrelle, CY, Huang, CC, Tsai,
       ST, Chen, KC, Huang, JS, Wong, TY, Lai, YH, Wu, YH, Hsueh,
       WT, Wu, SY, Yen, CJ, Chang, JY, Lin, CL, Weng, YL, Yang, HC,
       Chen, YS, and Chang, JS. 2019. "Oral Hygiene and the Overall

Survival of Head and Neck Cancer Patients." *Cancer Medicine*, No. 8: 1854–1864. https://doi.org/10.1002/cam4.2059

19.   Leung, SY, Chung, LP, Yuen, ST, Ho, CM, Wong, MP, and Chan, SY. 1995. "Lymphoepithelial Carcinoma of the Salivary Gland: In situ Detection of Epstein-Barr Virus." *Journal of Clinical Pathology*, No. 48: 1022–1027. https://doi.org/10.1136/jcp.48.11.1022

20.   Ribeiro, KB, Levi, JE, Pawlita, M, Koifman, S, Matos, E, Eluf-Neto, J, Wunsch-Filho, V, Curado, MP, Shangina, O, Zaridze, D, Szeszenia-Dabrowska, N, Lissowska, J, Daudt, A, Menezes, A, Bencko, V, Mates, D, Fernandez, L, Fabianova, E, Gheit, T, Tommasino, M, Boffetta, P, Brennan, P, and Waterboer, T. 2011. "Low Human Papillomavirus Prevalence in Head and Neck Cancer: Results from Two Large Case-Control Studies in High-Incidence Regions." *International Journal of Epidemiology*, No. 40: 489-502. https://doi.org/10.1093/ije/dyq249

21.   Dai, M, Clifford, GM, le Calvez, F, Castellsagué, X, Snijders, PJF, Pawlita, M, Herrero, R, Hainaut, P, and Franceschi, S. 2004. "Human Papillomavirus Type 16 and TP53 Mutation in Oral Cancer: Matched Analysis of the IARC Multicenter Study." *Cancer Research*, No. 64: 468–471. https://doi.org/10.1158/0008-5472.can-03-3284

22.   Park, DG, Woo, BH, Lee, BJ, Yoon, S, Cho, Y, Kim, Y-D, Park, HR, and Song, JM. 2019. "Serum Levels of Interleukin-6 and Titers of Antibodies against *Porphyromonas gingivalis* Could Be Potential Biomarkers for the Diagnosis of Oral Squamous Cell Carcinoma." *International Journal of Molecular Sciences*, No. 20: 2749. https://doi.org/10.3390/ijms20112749

23.   Hujoel, PP, Drangsholt, M, Spiekerman, C, and Weiss, NS. 2003. "An exploration of the Periodontitis-Cancer Association." *Annals of Epidemiology*, No. 13: 312–316. https://doi.org/10.1016/s1047-2797(02)00425-8

24.   Freudenheim, JL, Genco, RJ, LaMonte, MJ, Millen, AE, Hovey, KM, Mai, X, Nwizu, N, Andrews, CA, and Wactawski-Wende, J. 2016. "Periodontal Disease and Breast Cancer: Prospective Cohort Study of Postmenopausal Women." *Cancer Epidemiology, Biomarkers & Prevention*, No. 25 (1): 43–50.

25.   Shi, T, Min, M, Sun, C, Zhang, Y, Liang, M, and Sun, Y. 2018. "Periodontal Disease and Susceptibility to Breast Cancer: A Meta-analysis of Observational Studies." *Journal of Clinical Periodontology*, No. 45: 1025–1033. https://doi.org/10.1111/jcpe.12982

26.   Maisonneuve, P, Amar, S, and Lowenfels, AB. 2017. "Periodontal
       Disease, Edentulism, and Pancreatic Cancer: A Meta-analysis."
       Annals of Oncology, No. 28: 985–995.
       https://doi.org/10.1093/annonc/mdx019

27.   Stolzenberg-Solomon, RZ, Dodd, KW, Blaser, MJ, Virtamo, J,
       Taylor, PR, and Albanes, D. 2003. "Tooth Loss, Pancreatic Cancer,
       and *Helicobacter pylori*." *American Journal of Clinical Nutrition*,
       No. 78: 176–181. https://doi.org/10.1093/ajcn/78.1.176

28.   Michaud, DS, Izard, J, Wilhelm-Benartzi, CS, You, D-H, Grote, VA,
       Tjønneland, A, Dahm, CC, Overvad, K, Jenab, M, Fedirko, V,
       Boutron-Ruault, MC, Clavel-Chapelon, F, Racine, A, Kaaks, R,
       Boeing, H, Foerster, J, Trichopoulou, A, Lagiou, P, Trichopoulos, D,
       Sacerdote, C, Sieri, S, Palli, D, Tumino, R, Panico, S, Siersema, PD,
       Peeters, PHM, Lund, E, Barricarte, A, Huerta, J-M, Molina-Montes,
       E, Dorronsoro, M, Quirós, JR, Duell, EJ, Ye, W, Sund, M, Lindkvist,
       B, Johansen, D, Khaw, K-T, Wareham, N, Travis, RC, Vineis, P,
       Bueno-de-Mesquita, HB, and Riboli, E. 2013. "Plasma Antibodies
       to Oral Bacteria and Risk of Pancreatic Cancer in a Large European
       Prospective Cohort Study." *Gut*, No. 62: 1764–1770.
       https://doi.org/10.1136/gutjnl-2012-303006

29.   Ahn, J, Segers, S, and Hayes, RB. 2012. "Periodontal Disease,
       Porphyromonas gingivalis Serum Antibody Levels and Orodigestive
       Cancer Mortality." *Carcinogenesis*, No. 33: 1055–1058.
       https://doi.org/10.1093/carcin/bgs112

30.   Wu, Y, Shi, X, Li, Y, Shi, X, Xia, J, Gu, Y, Qian Q, and Hong Y.
       2020. "Hematopoietic and Lymphatic Cancers in Patients with
       Periodontitis: A Systematic Review and Meta-analysis." *Medicina
       Oral, Patologia Oral, Cirugia Bucal*, No. 25: e21–e28.
       https://doi.org/10.4317/medoral.23166

CHAPTER 12

RHEUMATOID ARTHRITIS

Rheumatic disorders are a group of conditions characterized by the presence of a high degree of circulating autoantibodies in the patient's blood. Periodontitis has been associated with some conditions constituting rheumatoid disorders. This chapter explores rheumatoid arthritis (RA), but other rheumatic diseases that produce oral symptoms include Sjögren syndrome and Behçet's disease. Only a few scientific studies link oral infections to gout, lupus, spondyloarthropathies, systemic sclerosis, or infectious arthritis.

Rheumatoid arthritis

RA is an autoimmune disease of unclear aetiology. It is characterized by synovial joint inflammation progressing to cartilage and bone destruction and causing much discomfort. Symmetrical pain from several joints is characteristic. There is no cure for RA; hence, limiting pain and discomfort is important to maintain optimal joint function. A hypothesis of a link between RA and PD has been put forward (1–6). The syndrome is three times more common in women and affects only a small proportion of the population, estimated to be 1.0% to 3.0% (7).

Periodontitis and RA are both chronic inflammatory diseases and both are multifactorial. They share common disease-progressing factors, such as osteoclasia, human leukocyte antigen-DR4 allelic genes, an immunological profile, and characteristic cytokines. Proinflammatory mediators have the ability to break down synovial membranes and periodontium around teeth. Both diseases are characterized by anticitrullinated protein antibodies (ACPAs) and anti-α-enolase. In addition, antibodies to one of the oral pathogens of periodontitis, Pg, have been isolated from synovial joints in RA (8). Two approaches have been used: studying clinical periodontal status information and ACPA level, the diagnostic parameter for RA.

Prevalence of rheumatoid arthritis

A major diagnostic factor in RA is ACPA level. Van Zanten, Arends, Roozendaal, Limburg, Maas et al. studied the prevalence of ACPAs in the large Lifelines cohort of 40,136 participants in the Netherlands (9). The persons were mainly of Caucasian origin. ACPA levels ≥ 6.2 U/ml were considered positive. The authors included demographic and clinical information on smoking, PD, and symptoms of musculoskeletal disease. RA was defined by self-reported RA, relevant medication, and a medical specialist visit in the previous year. In all, 401 (1%) persons had ACPA levels ≥ 6.2 U/ml. Among persons without RA were 0.8% persons with ACPA-positive levels. The ACPA-positive level was associated with older age, women, smoking, joint complaints, and RA-positive first-degree family members. In non-RA cases, age, smoking, and joint complaints were more frequent in ACPA-positive participants than in ACPA-negative participants.

Prevalence of periodontitis in rheumatoid arthritis cases

Eriksson, Nise, Kats, Luttropp et al. investigated the prevalence of periodontitis in RA cases in the Swedish Epidemiological Investigation of Rheumatoid Arthritis, including 2,740 RA cases and 3,942 matched controls in their analyses (1). This constituted a population-based case-control cohort. The authors also used data from the National Dental Health Registry and quality assured a sample for periodontal diagnoses. The authors concluded there was no increased prevalence of periodontitis in patients with RA compared to healthy controls or any differences in ACPA or rheumatoid factor (RF) status among patients with RA. Smoking and age were risk factors for periodontitis both in patients with RA and healthy controls.

Arkema, Karlson, and Costenbader also observed this lack of association between periodontitis/oral health parameters and RA in a large study on American women (N = 81,132 participants, including 292 RA cases) (10). The researchers did not find any significant associations of RA with periodontal surgery (RR = 1.24, 95% CI 0.83–1.83), tooth loss (RR = 1.18, 95% CI 0.47–2.95), or periodontal surgery and tooth extractions combined.

Mikuls, Thiele, Deane, Payne et al. studied RA prevalence in cross-sectional studies by comparing two groups in their ongoing prospective cohort study in the US – Studies of the Etiology of Rheumatoid Arthritis. The aim of this study was to investigate genetic and epidemiologic associations for RA-related autoimmunity in a preclinical RA period (11). One group was a cohort of patients with the HLA-DRA allele, the allele diagnostic of RA (n = 113; a high-risk group, n = 38), and the other group was a cohort with persons of first-degree relatives of patients with RA (n = 171). Mikuls, Thiele, Deane, Payne et al. were interested in studying the relationship between autoantibodies to RA, RF, and antibodies of oral bacteria (Pg, Pi, and Fn). The researchers found that elevated levels of antibodies to Pg but not Pi or Fn was associated with RA-related autoantibodies in persons at risk of RA. The authors concluded that this "supports the hypothesis that PG [*Porphyromonas gingivalis*] infection may play a central role in the early loss of tolerance to self-antigens in RA pathogenesis."

Treatment of periodontitis in rheumatoid arthritis cases

From this evidence, the question of effect PD treatment on patients with RA arises. Local periodontal treatment is certain to have some effect on the oral cavity, but does this extend to improving RA symptoms? Such a study is reported from Turkey (3). Erciyas, Sezer, Ustün, Pehlivan et al. established a prospective cohort study of 30 patients with RA and moderate-to-high disease activity (disease activity score [DAS] 28 ≥ 3.2) and chronic periodontitis and compared the group to 30 patients with low disease activity (DAS28 < 3.2) and chronic periodontitis. DAS28 is a measure of disease activity used for patients with DA. Erciyas, Sezer, Ustün, Pehlivan et al. explored clinical periodontal measurements and systemic inflammatory parameters, such as erythrocyte sedimentation rate, CRP, TNF-α, DAS28, and periodontal parameters. At the three-month evaluation, the researchers found a reduction in RA severity as measured by erythrocyte sedimentation rate, CRP, TNF-α in serum, and DAS28 in patients with mildly or moderately to highly active RA registered with chronic periodontitis.

Fisher, Cartwright, Quirke, de Pablo et al. investigated whether ACPAs were associated with peptidylarginine deiminase (PPAD) expressed by Pg (4). The authors conducted a nested case-control study to study the prediction of RA using smoking and the role of Pg. Four populations of the European Prospective Investigation into Cancer and Nutrition study were included. Each pre-RA case (n = 103) was matched with three controls. ACPAs can be identified years before RA diagnosis. Smoking is a risk factor for RA and periodontitis. Fisher, Cartwright, Quirke, de Pablo et al. concluded that smoking was a risk factor for RA before its onset. However, they did not find that Pg was associated with pre-RA autoimmunity or that it inferred RA risk in the early phases before disease onset. Hence, they concluded that antibodies to PPAD peptides were not an early feature of ACPA ontogeny.

Terao, Asai, Hashimoto, Yamazaki et al. in Japan, analysed data from 9,554 healthy persons (12). ACPA and IgM RF were measured. Their periodontal status was assessed by the number of missing teeth, community periodontal index, and degree of loss of attachment level of the teeth. All three PD parameters were significantly associated with ACPA but not RF. This finding was also found in nonsmokers (n = 6,206). The study supports an association between PD and RA but does not explain the direct linkage.

Microbiology and immunology

Silvestre-Rangil, Bagán, Silvestre, and Bagán prospectively studied 73 patients with RA and 73 control persons (5). The researchers examined periodontal pocket depth, CAL, bleeding index, PI, DMFT index of periodontal status, and salivary flow status. Differences in periodontal status was observed, as patients with RA had more severe symptoms of periodontitis and tended to suffer from decreased salivary rate. The latter predisposes to periodontitis and caries. Sjögren syndrome was not diagnosed.

A link between RA and periodontitis is the ACPAs in RA cases (2). Among oral bacteria, Pg expresses the enzyme PPAD, which can generate citrillinated proteins and peptides. Citrullination or deamination is the conversion of the amino acid arginine in a protein into the amino acid citrulline. Citrulline, however, is not one of the 20 amino acids of DNA; it is a result of a posttranslational modification. Wegner, N, Wait, R, Sroka, A, Eick, S, Nguyen et al claim that their result provides "a novel model where Pg-mediated citrullination of bacterial and host proteins provides a molecular mechanism for generating antigens that drive the autoimmune response in RA." Eleven bacterial species were tested, and Pg was the only one believed to trigger the immune response in RA. The tested species were *Porphyromonas gingivalis, Fusobacterium nucleatum, Aggregatibacter actinomycetemcomitans, Prevotella intermedia, Prevotella oralis, Capnocytophaga gingivalis, Capnocytophaga ochracea, Streptococcus constellatus, S. gordonii, S. sanguinis,* and *S. salivarius.*

Äyräväinen, Leirisalo-Repo, M, Kuuliala, A, Ahola et al. conducted a prospective study of an association between RA and oral health parameters in Helsinki, Finland, with about nine years of follow-up (13). Fifty-three patients with early-stage RA (ERA) taking disease-modifying antirheumatic drugs (DMARDs), 28 patients with chronic RA (CRA) with poor response to conventional DMARDs, and 43 matched controls were included in the study. After baseline, patients with ERA started synthetic DMARDs, and those with CRA started biological DMARDs. Moderate periodontitis was more frequent in patients with RA than controls (67.3% vs 39.5%). In addition, the researchers found Pg to be more prevalent in patients with ERA than in patients with CRA or controls. The antirheumatic drugs did not seem to affect the results of the study.

Possible linkage between oral infection and RA have been shown in SRs of studies involving clinical risk measurements. Fuggle, Smith, Kaul, and Sofat included 21 studies (N = 153,492 participants) that met their inclusion criteria, of which 17 compared patients with RA to healthy controls and 4 compared the first group to patients with osteoarthritis (n = 1,378 participants) (14). The clinical measurements mean probing depth, BOP, or absolute value of CAL were raised. The result for patients with RA versus healthy controls was an RR of 1.13 (95% CI 1.04–1.23, p = 0.006), but there was a great degree of heterogeneity between the studies (I^2 = 95%). BOP risk was greater in patients with osteoarthritis than in patients with RA.

Concluding remarks

The studies mentioned in this chapter do not provide any causal conclusions regarding oral infection and RA. Treatment of periodontal infection in RA reduces common inflammatory parameters.

References

1.   Eriksson, K, Nise, L, Kats, A, Luttropp, E, Catrina, AI, Askling, J, Jansso, L, Alfredsson, L, Klareskog, L, Lundberg, K, and Yucel-Lindberg, T. 2016. "Prevalence of Periodontitis in Patients with Established Rheumatoid Arthritis: A Swedish Population Based Case-Control Study.: *PLoS One*, No. 11: e0155956.
2.   Wegner, N, Wait, R, Sroka, A, Eick, S, Nguyen, K-A, Lundberg, K, Kinloch, A, Culshaw, S, Potempa, J, and Venables, PJ. 2010. "Peptidylarginine Deiminase from *Porphyromonas gingivalis* Citrullinates Human Fibrinogen and α-enolase: Implications for Autoimmunity in Rheumatoid Arthritis." *Arthritis & Rheumatology*, No. 62: 72.
3.   Erciyas, K, Sezer, U, Ustün, K, Pehlivan, Y, Kisacik, B, Senyurt, SZ, Tarakçioğlu, M, and Onat, AM. 2013. "Effects of Periodontal Therapy on Disease Activity and Systemic Inflammation in Rheumatoid Arthritis Patients." *Oral Diseases*, No. 19: 394–400.
4.   Fisher, BA, Cartwright, AJ, Quirke, A-M, de Pablo, P, Romaguera, D, Panico, S, Mattiello, A, Gavrila, D, Navarro, C, Sacerdote, C,

Vineis, P, Tumino, R, Lappin, DF, Apatzidou, D, Culshaw, S, Potempa, J, Michaud, DS, Riboli, E, and Venables, PJ. 2015. "Smoking, *Porphyromonas gingivalis* and the Immune Response to Citrullinated Autoantigens before the Clinical Onset of Rheumatoid Arthritis in a Southern European Nested Case-Control Study." *BMC Musculoskeletal Disorders*, No. 16: 331.

5. Silvestre-Rangil, J, Bagán, L, Silvestre, FJ, and Bagán, JV. 2016. "Oral Manifestations of Rheumatoid Arthritis. A Cross-Sectional Study of 73 Patients." *Clinical Oral Investigations*, No. 20: 2575–2580.

6. Li, R, Tian, C, Postlethwaite, A, Jiao, Y, Garcia-Godoy, F, Pattanaik D, Wei, D, Gu, W, and Li, J. 2017. "Rheumatoid Arthritis and Periodontal Disease: What Are the Similarities and Differences?" *International Journal of Rheumatic Diseases*, No. 20: 1887–1901.

7. Kaur, S, White, S, and Bartold, M. 2012. "Periodontal Disease as a Risk Factor for Rheumatoid Arthritis: A Systematic Review." *JBI Library of Systematic Reviews*, No. 10 (42 Suppl): 1–12. https://doi.org/10.11124/jbisrir-2012-288

8. Fiorillo, L, Cervino, G, Laino, L, D'Amico, C, Mauceri, R, Tozum, TF, Gaeta, M, and Cicciù, M. 2019. "*Porphyromonas gingivalis*, Periodontal and Systemic Implications: A Systematic Review." *Dentistry Journal (Basel)*, No. 7: 114. https://doi.org/10.3390/dj7040114

9. van Zanten, A, Arends, S, Roozendaal, C, Limburg, PC, Maas, F, Trouw, LA· Toes, REM· Huizinga, TWJ, Bootsma, H· and Brouwer, E. 2017. "Presence of Anticitrullinated Protein Antibodies in a Large Population-Based Cohort from the Netherlands." *Annals of the Rheumatic Diseases*, No. 76: 1184 1190.

10. Arkema, EV, Karlson, EW, and Costenbader, KH. 2010. "A Prospective Study of Periodontal Disease and Risk of Rheumatoid Arthritis." *Journal of Rheumatology*, No. 37: 1800–1804.

11. Mikuls, TR, Thiele, GM, Deane, KD, Payne, JB, O'Dell, JR, Yu, F, Sayles, H, Weisman, MW, Gregersen, PK, Buckner, JH, Keating, RM, Derber, LA, Robinson, WH, Holers, VM, and Norris, JM. 2012. "*Porphyromonas gingivalis* and Disease-Related Autoantibodies in Individuals at Increased Risk of Rheumatoid Arthritis." *Arthritis & Rheumatology*, No. 64: 3522–3530.

12. Terao, C, Asai, K, Hashimoto, M, Yamazaki, T, Ohmura, K, Yamaguchi, A, Takahashi, K, Takei, N, Ishii, T, Kawaguchi, T, Tabara, Y, Takahashi, M, Nakayama, T, Kosugi, S, Sekine, A, Fujii, T, Yamada, R, Mimori, T, Matsuda, F, Bessho, K, and Nagahama

Study Group. 2015. "Significant Association of Periodontal Disease with Anti-citrullinated Peptide Antibody in a Japanese Healthy Population - the Nagahama Study." *Journal of Autoimmunity*, No. 59: 85–90.

13.   Äyräväinen, L, Leirisalo-Repo, M, Kuuliala, A, Ahola, K, Koivuniemi, R, Meurman, JH, and Heikkinen, AM. 2017. "Periodontitis in Early and Chronic Rheumatoid Arthritis: A Prospective Follow-Up Study in Finnish Population." *BMJ Open*, No. 7: e011916.

14.   Fuggle, NR, Smith, TO, Kaul, A, and Sofat, N. 2016. "Hand to Mouth: A Systematic Review and Meta-analysis of the Association between Rheumatoid Arthritis and Periodontitis." *Frontiers in Immunology*, No. **7**: 80.

CHAPTER 13

PREGNANCY AND PRETERM BIRTH

Pregnancy, although not a systemic disease, is an important condition, and adverse infections such as periodontitis and caries ought not to occur during the pregnancy period. Several studies have been conducted to understand the possible association between oral infections and adverse pregnancy outcomes. If the pathological mechanisms of how and why oral infections occur could be identified, then women can be advised on how to prevent such infections. How strong is the evidence of an association? Two possible pathways have been identified to explain this association: first, the direct path in which oral bacteria and/or bacterial products act on the foetal-placental unit (1), and second, the indirect path in which microbes and inflammatory mediators circulate and impact the foetal-placental unit. According to the third EFP/AAP report from 2013, periodontal therapy is safe and leads to better periodontal health of pregnant women (1).

Periodontal disease in pregnancy

Niederman conducted an SR of observational data comprising 14 cohort and 19 cross sectional studies to explore GI and/or BOP in pregnant women (2). The results showed that GI was lowest in the first trimester but increased in the second and third trimesters. Furthermore, postpartum values of GI were lower than those of the second and third trimesters. Small changes in plaque levels were reported in these studies. These observational results indicate but do not prove a causal relationship between GI score and pregnancy; nevertheless, pregnant women can benefit from paying attention to oral health. Nonpregnant women had a lower GI value than women in the 2nd and 3rd terms of pregnancy.

Periodontal treatment in pregnancy

It is important to conduct intervention trials/RCTs to study the effect of periodontal treatment. If the treatment under investigation has an effect, then pregnant women ought to be advised to have a dental examination and undergo the necessary treatment. Bi, Emami, Luo, Santamaria et al. conducted an SR in 2019 to assess the effect of periodontal treatment during pregnancy on maternal, foetal, and neonatal outcomes (3). Studies on perinatal mortality and maternal and neonatal morbidity were searched, and 20 RCTs of periodontal treatment versus control with a total of 8,171 study participants were included. Their primary outcome of perinatal mortality among 5,942 participants was significantly reduced by RR = 0.53 (0.30–0.93, p = 0.03, I^2 = 0%). The study also found a reduced risk of preterm births (n = 7,335; RR = 0.78 [0.62–0.98], p = 0.03, I^2 = 72%). There was a high degree of heterogeneity among the included studies. Periodontal treatment during pregnancy was found to significantly increase the birthweight of the babies. Preeclampsia, GDM, caesarean section, small for gestational age, or congenital malformations were not affected by periodontal treatment.

Gestational diabetes mellitus

First-time onset of diabetes in pregnancy is termed gestational diabetes mellitus (GDM), and this condition could put the mother and foetus at risk of serious complications. Although the aetiology is not well understood, glucose intolerance is an underlying factor. Because periodontitis has implications for the immune system, a possible association has been investigated in several studies. In an SR, Lima, Cyrino, Dutra, Oliveira da Silveira et al. (2016) identified 190 studies to determine if periodontal treatment during pregnancy could reduce the risk of GDM and included 8 in their review (4). The analysis of four cross-sectional studies showed an OR of 1.67 (1.20–2.32), while the OR of the case-control studies was 2.66 (1.52–4.65). The authors noted that the studies were heterogenic; hence, they were careful about concluding that there is a positive association between periodontitis and GDM. Abariga and Whitcomb conducted an SR and included 10 studies according to their inclusion criteria (5). Diagnostic criteria varied for GDM and periodontitis, causing some heterogeneity between the studies. The studies included 5,724 participants, while 624 were cases. The overall result of the meta-analysis to assess if periodontitis was associated with GDM was 66% (OR = 1.66 [1.17–2.36], p < 0.05), I^2 = 50.5%. Subgroup analysis of case-control studies of 1,176 participants, including 380 cases, gave an OR of 1.85 (1.03–3.32, p < 0.05, I^2 = 68.4%). The OR of confounder adjusted results was 2.08 (1.21–3.58, p = 0.009, I^2 = 36.9%). The elevated I^2 reveals the need for prospective studies with more homogenous criteria for the diagnoses of periodontitis and diabetes.

Preeclampsia

In 2020, Konopka and Zakrzewska published an SR of cohort and RCT studies on PD and incidence of preeclampsia (6). The review found an association in four of six cohort studies, which included 2,724 pregnant women and 195 had preeclampsia. In three RCTs of nonsurgical treatment (SRP), the preventive effect of the intervention was not observed. The intervention group had 1,825 women, while the control group had 1,827 women. Preeclampsia was diagnosed equally in the two groups – with 116 in each, constituting 6.30% and 6.35%, respectively.

Preterm birth and birthweight

Microbiological indicators

Boggess, Moss, Madianos, Murtha et al. (2005) designed a prospective study that examined umbilical blood for factors of immune response and oral pathogens (7). Specimens from 640 births were examined, of which 48 (7%) were preterm. Cord serum levels of CRP, IL-1beta, IL-6, TNF-α, prostaglandin E2, and 8-isoprostane were measured by ELISA, which provides accurate measurements by the level of optical readings. This prospectively designed study showed that the presence of foetal IgM antibodies that fight against oral bacteria (p = 0.04), and infection parameters as high as the level of 8-isoprostane of TNF-α were higher in preterm births. The risk for preterm birth was increased by inflammatory parameters such as detectable CRP, or high 8-isoprostane, prostaglandin E2, or TNF-α.

Periodontal treatment

Using RCTs, a Cochrane report from 2017 reported evidence of the effect of periodontal treatment on a pregnant woman versus when there was no periodontal treatment during pregnancy (8). In all, 15 RCTs met their inclusion criteria for the meta-analyses. Eleven studies with 5,671 participants looked at preterm birth < 37 weeks, and the meta-analysis showed a nonsignificant difference (RR = 0.87, 95% CI 0.70–1.10). There was no indication at < 35 weeks. Seven studies with 3,470 participants examined the effect of periodontal treatment and the effect of birthweight < 2,500 g. The 9.7% reduction in the low birthweight category with periodontal treatment versus 12.6% without treatment was significant (RR = 0.67, 95% CI 0.48–0.95) except for birthweight < 1,500 g. Perinatal mortality for different periodontal treatments was compared, but the quality of evidence was very low. For either of the outcomes, maternal mortality and adverse effects of the intervention did not occur in any of the studies. The authors concluded that it is not clear if periodontal treatment during pregnancy has an impact on preterm birth (low-quality evidence). There is low-quality evidence that periodontal treatment may reduce low birthweight ($< 2,500$ g); hence, the confidence in the effect estimate is limited. There is insufficient evidence to determine the periodontal treatment that is better in preventing adverse obstetric outcomes.

Bi et al., as mentioned, found a reduced risk of preterm births among women who received periodontal treatment during pregnancy. ($n = 7,335$; RR = 0.78 (0.62–0.98), p = 0.03, I^2 = 72%) (there was a high degree of heterogeneity among the included studies) (3). It was also found that periodontal treatment during pregnancy significantly increased birthweight among women.

Govindasamy, Periyasamy, Narayanan, Balaji et al. published a review in 2020 that included 19 RCTs and concluded that periodontal therapy was beneficial to the oral health of pregnant women, but the studies did not show convincing benefits for the foetus (9). The difference in risk rates was large between the studies. The rate for preterm birth ranged from 0% to 53.5% for those having periodontal therapy versus controls (6.4%–72%). The rate for low birthweight for periodontal therapy was 0%–36% and 1.2%–53.9% for the controls. There was a large variation in the study results. The authors concluded that it can be inferred that nonsurgical therapy is safe during pregnancy and can be recommended as a part of antenatal care.

Concluding remarks

Periodontal treatment in pregnant women was not shown to affect preeclampsia in treated versus nontreated women, but an association with GDM was observed. There were variations in the study results regarding the effect on preterm birth or low birthweight but benefit regarding reduced perinatal mortality. Treatment of oral infections is of benefit to pregnant women, as concluded in the third EFP/AAP report from 2013 (1). Recent SRs do not change this conclusion.

References

1.   Sanz, M, Kornman, K, and Working Group 3 of the Joint EFP/AAP Workshop. 2013. "Periodontitis and adverse Pregnancy Outcomes:

Consensus Report of the Joint EFP/AAP Workshop on Periodontitis and Systemic Diseases." *Journal of Periodontology*, No. 84 (4 Suppl): S164–S169. https://doi.org/10.1902/jop.2013.1340016

2. Niederman, R. 2013. "Pregnancy Gingivitis and Causal Inference." *Evidence-Based Dentistry*, No. 14 (4): 107–108. https://doi.org/10.1038/sj.ebd.6400966

3. Bi, WG, Emami, E, Luo, Z-C, Santamaria, C, and Wei, SQ. 2019. "Effect of Periodontal Treatment in Pregnancy on Perinatal Outcomes: A Systematic Review and Meta-analysis." *Journal of Maternal-Fetal and Neonatal Medicine*. 34 (19): 3259-3268. https://doi.org/10.1080/14767058.2019.1678142

4. Lima, RFE, Cyrino, RM, Dutra, B de C, Oliveira da Silveira, J, Martins, CC, Cota, LOM, and Costa, FO. 2016. "Association between Periodontitis and Gestational Diabetes Mellitus: Systematic Review and Meta-analysis." *Journal of Periodontology*, No. 87 (1): 48–57. https://doi.org/10.1902/jop.2015.150311

5. Abariga, SA, and Whitcomb, BW. 2016. "Periodontitis and Gestational Diabetes Mellitus: A Systematic Review and Meta-analysis of Observational Studies." *BMC Pregnancy Childbirth*, No. 16 (1): 344. https://doi.org/10.1186/s12884-016-1145-z

6. Konopka, T, and Zakrzewska, A. 2020. "Periodontitis and Risk for Preeclampsia - a Systematic Review." *Ginekologia Polska*, No. 91 (3): 158–164. https://doi.org/10.5603/GP.2020.0024

7. Boggess, KA, Moss, K, Madianos, P, Murtha, AP, Beck, J, and Offenbacher, S. 2005. "Fetal Immune Response to Oral Pathogens and Risk of Preterm Birth." *American Journal of Obstetrics and Gynecology*, No. 193 (3 Pt 2): 1121–1126. https://doi.org/10.1016/j.ajog.2005.05.050

8. Iheozor-Ejiofor, Z, Middleton, P, Esposito, M, and Glenny, A-M. 2017. "Treating Periodontal Disease for Preventing Adverse Birth Outcomes in Pregnant Women." *Cochrane Database of Systematic Reviews*, No. 6 (6): CD005297. https://doi.org/10.1002/14651858.CD005297.pub3

9. Govindasamy, R, Periyasamy, S, Narayanan, M, Balaji, VR, Dhanasekaran, M, and Karthikeyan, B. 2020. "The Influence of Nonsurgical Periodontal Therapy on the Occurrence of Adverse Pregnancy Outcomes: A Systematic Review of the Current Evidence." *Journal of Indian Society of Periodontology*, No. 24 (1): 7–14. https://doi.org/10.4103/jisp.jisp_228_19

CHAPTER 14

ALZHEIMER'S DISEASE

Alzheimers disease (AD) is a serious form of dementia, and it was first recognized and described by Alois Alzheimer. The first case was reported in 1907; however, there is still no cure, nor is the direct cause known. The WHO recognizes AD as an increasing public health priority (1). With the increasing longevity of many populations, this disease may be more common and potentially become a burden on many health facilities worldwide, as well as on afflicted individuals and families. In short, AD is a serious form of dementia that is progressive and causes cognitive impairment that impacts daily living and activities for women and men. It is a cause of disability, morbidity, and mortality in the elderly. A rare genetic form may arise in middle age, but most cases occur late in life. Late-onset AD (LOAD) is believed to be caused by an interplay between genes and environmental factors. The effect of several factors (such as infections, educational level, physical exercise, vascular factors, and other factors) on AD has been examined, but none is conclusive. The genetic picture is becoming clearer. The main pathophysiologic changes in the brain include amyloid plaques and neurofibrillary tangles (NFTs), which characterize AD. These pathologic changes lead to different forms of neuronal degeneration and further develop into macroscopic atrophy. Thus far, AD diagnosis is based on clinical parameters, biologic markers, and pathologic changes observed on MRI scans.

Much research is ongoing to elucidate causal factors that can lead to the development of future appropriate treatment options. One of the factors being investigated is oral infection. Olsen and Singhrao has written a comprehensive review of possible pathological pathways (such as genetics), including those originating from oral infections, and reported a possible causal pathologic mechanism (2). The pathological hallmarks of AD are numerous extracellular amyloid beta (Aβ) plaques and intraneuronal NFTs. They distinguish between an intrinsic model and an extrinsic model of pathology. The intrinsic model is based on the blood-brain barrier being intact and that neuroinflammation occurs by inflammatory elements of AD pathology and inappropriate activation of the complement system in association with Aβ, Aβ plaques, and NFTs. The extrinsic model accounts for the ability of glial cells to communicate through the vascular system, meeting the immune challenges of elements from bacterial infections. This is possible as the circumventricular organs and the choroid plexus are devoid of the blood-brain barrier.

Several bacteria, bacterial products, and inflammation markers have been investigated (3). Infectious agents include oral or nonoral *Treponema* spp., as well as viruses such as herpes simplex virus type 1, which is known to be dormant in cerebral nerve ganglia or yeasts (*Candida* spp.). Inflammatory markers include CRP and IL-1. The infectious route can be initiated by periodontal infection, which can be directly transmitted through the blood to the brain or by bacterial products that stimulate immunological reactions and cause changes in the brain. Maintaining a healthy periodontium is, therefore, important. Further research is needed to fully understand the cause of LOAD to develop prevention strategies and targeted treatment.

Gatz, Mortimer, Fratiglioni, Johansson et al. investigated the risk of developing AD due to tooth loss in identical twins in the Swedish Twin Registry (4). Twins aged 65 years or more and alive in 1998 were included in the study. They were all screened for different parameters, including dementia assessment and tooth loss. A case-control study design involving 310 persons with dementia and 3,063 nondemented persons was used. In all, 106 monozygotic twins were discordant for dementia. The researchers found that tooth loss around 35 years of age or earlier resulted in an OR of 1.74 (95% CI 1.35–2.24) for developing AD. The risk factors had been assessed independently 30 years earlier. The results indicate that an inflammatory load contributes to AD risk.

Using the Nun Study (US), Stein, Desrosiers, Donegan, Yepes et al. linked periodontitis to cognitive deficit and proposed PD as a risk factor for developing AD later in life (5). Ten annual cognitive assessments of 144 participants (75–98 years) were available. Neuropathologic autopsy findings were available for the 118 participants who died during follow-up. Stein, Desrosiers, Donegan, Yepes et al. found that persons with the lowest number of teeth had the highest prevalence and incidence of dementia.

Singhrao and Olsen further assessed oral infections as causative factors of AD (6). They investigated the literature on Pg and possible association with AD and reported studies that used mouse models with oral infections caused by Pg or introduction of its LPS caused neurological lesions, indicating dementia. A range of signs and symptoms were reported as extracellular Aβ plaques, phosphorylated tau, NFTs, widespread acute and chronic inflammation, and blood-brain barrier defects, along with the clinical phenotype showing impaired learning and spatial memory. Progressive cognitive impairment sufficient to impact on activities of daily living – is a major cause of dependence, disability and mortality.

In 2021, Olsen and Singhrao put forward arguments for an association between the level of lactoferrin in saliva and AD (7). It has been reported that reduced levels of salivary lactoferrin can be a plausible biomarker for Aβ accumulation in brains with AD. Olsen and Singhrao discussed whether a low level of lactoferrin in saliva may influence the development of oral dysbiosis, indicating a link between these two factors.

Concluding remarks

This overview shows that studies exploring the association between oral health and AD have been carried out, but the long induction time and the development of the disease makes conducting these studies demanding. Research is ongoing on many frontiers of medicine and dentistry to understand the aetiology and progress of the disease. Oral infections have inherent pathologic effects that are important to study in relation to AD.

References

1.   Lane, CA, Hardy, J, and Schott, JM. 2018. "Alzheimer's Disease." *European Journal of Neurology*, No. 25: 59–70.
2.   Olsen, I, and Singhrao SK. 2015. "Can Oral Infection Be a Risk Factor for Alzheimer's Disease?" *Journal of Oral Microbiology*, No. 7: 29143.
3.   Dewhirst, FE, Chen, T, Izard, J, Paster, BJ, Tanner, AC, Yu, WH, Lakshmanan, A, and Wade, WG. 2010. "The Human Oral Microbiome." *Journal of Bacteriology*, No. 192: 5002–5017.
4.   Gatz, M, Mortimer, JA, Fratiglioni, L, Johansson, B, Berg, S, Reynolds, CA, and Pedersen, NL. 2006. "Potentially Modifiable Risk Factors for Dementia in Identical Twins." *Alzheimer's & Dementia*, No. 2: 110–117.
5.   Stein, PS, Desrosiers, M, Donegan, SJ, Yepes, JF, and Kryscio, RJ. 2007. "Tooth Loss, Dementia and Neuropathology in the Nun Study." *Journal of the American Dental Association*, No. 138: 1314–1322.

6.   Singhrao, SK, and Olsen, I. 2019. "Assessing the Role of *Porphyromonas gingivalis* in Periodontitis to Determine a Causative Relationship with Alzheimer's Disease." *Journal of Oral Microbiology*, No. 11: 1563405.

7.   Olsen, I, and Singhrao, SK. 2021. "Low Levels of Salivary Lactoferrin May Affect Oral Dysbiosis and Contribute to Alzheimer's Disease: A Hypothesis." *Medical Hypotheses*, No. 146: 110393.

CHAPTER 15

GASTRIC ULCER

A large cross-sectional study in Korea studied the association between self-reported periodontitis and chronic gastritis/peptic ulcer. The Korean Genome and Epidemiology Study (2004–2016) provided data on 173,209 participants: 9,983 with periodontitis and 125,336 with no periodontitis (1). The adjusted OR of periodontitis increasing the risk of chronic gastritis and peptic ulcer was 2.22 (2.10–2.34, $p < 0.001$) and 1.86 (1.74–1.98, $p < 0.001$), respectively.

Concluding remarks

Epidemiologic studies on gastric ulcer and oral infection are limited. However, this study from South Korea is large, and the estimates are of reasonable size with narrow CIs.

References

1. Byun, SH, Min, C, Hong, SJ, Choi, HG, and Koh, DH. 2020. "Analysis of the Relation between Periodontitis and Chronic Gastritis/Peptic Ulcer: A Cross-Sectional Study Using KoGES HEXA Data." *International Journal of Environmental Research and Public Health*, No. 17 (12): 4387. https://doi.org/10.3390/ijerph17124387

CHAPTER 16

INFECTIONS OF THE FACE AND NECK

If untreated, infections can spread. From the oral cavity, there can be several reasons for local spread of infections to adjoining structures and rarely descending to the mediastinum or through the intraorbital route to the cavernous sinuses of the brain.

Acute infections observed as abscess or cellulitis of the head and neck may be of oral origin. A differential diagnosis should include an oral examination in such cases to provide the best treatment. These infections may be superficial, deep, or extended downwards to the mediastinum (1). Superficial infections may be in the intraorbital region, maxillary and mandibular regions, infratemporal fossa, masseteric space, and pterygomandibular space. Deep infections extend into the sublingual spaces, the lateral pharyngeal space, the retropharyngeal space, the carotid bundle, Ludwig's angina, cavernous sinus thrombosis, and thrombophlebitis. The close proximity of the teeth to the maxillary sinuses allows for the spread of infection through the maxilla, and osteomyelitis may also occur.

References

1.   Farmer and Lawton eds. 1966. *Stones' Oral and Dental Diseases*. 5th ed. Edinburgh: E. & S. Livingstone.

PART 3:

ORAL SIGNS AND SYMPTOMS OF SYSTEMIC DISEASES

CHAPTER 17

THE IMPACT OF SYSTEMIC DISEASES ON ORAL HEALTH

The first clinical trial

A well-known study, considered the first clinical trial, was carried out on a ship in 1747. The doctor on board – James Lind (1716–1794), a Scottish doctor – noticed that many of the crew on board suffered badly from what was known as scurvy, which was caused by a lack of vitamin C in the diet. Gingival bleeding was a major symptom, in addition to anaemia, other sores, headache, toothache, tooth loss, and chest pain. Since the 17th century, it has been known that citrus fruits can protect against scurvy.

On long voyages across the oceans at that time, the crew needed to be fit and healthy, not lying sick in bed. Scurvy was known, but no treatment was available. Dr Lind decided to test six different treatments in one of the first studies registered, which is quite similar to today's clinical trials: 'I chose twelve patients with scurvy on board the HMS Salisbury during the voyage. The patients were as similar as I could get them and had a common diet.'

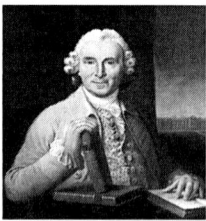

Figure 1. James Lind (1747)

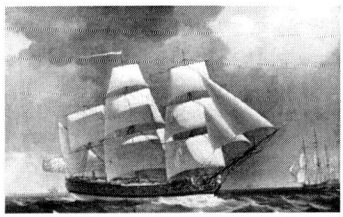

Figure 2. HMS Salisbury

Lind thought that scurvy was due to putrefaction of the body, which could be prevented by acids. Thus, he chose to experiment with dietary supplements of acidic quality. In his experiment, he divided 12 scorbutic sailors into 6 groups and gave them all the same diet. In addition, the following was given to the groups: Group 1 was given a quart of cider daily; Group 2, 25 drops of elixir of vitriol (sulfuric acid); Group 3, six spoonsful of vinegar; Group 4, half a pint of seawater; Group 5, two oranges and one lemon; and Group 6, a spicy paste plus a drink of barley water. Group 5's treatment stopped after six days when they ran out of fruit. However, by that time, one sailor was fit for duty, and the other had almost recovered. Apart from that, only Group 1 improved.

Dr Lind continued working for the improvement of hygiene in the Royal Navy and further influenced preventive medicine and improved nutrition. Today, scurvy is rare.

Systemic conditions with oral symptoms

Systemic disorders of known and unknown aetiology are related to secondary oral infections or other symptoms due to ulcerations in part or of the entire oral mucosa. Oral symptoms by themselves are challenging to manage, as they can cause painful lesions and lead to masticatory problems. However, they are important adjuncts to the differential diagnosis of the underlying systemic disease (1–3). In this respect, dentists can assist in diagnosis and coordinate the diagnosis and treatment with the patient's physician as needed. In 2018, Porter, Mercadante, and Fedele wrote a useful overview of the many systemic conditions that have oral symptoms (1). They focussed on systemic diseases that affect the oral mucosa, including white lesions and salivary glands.

Aphthous ulcers

Aphthous ulcers appear spontaneously and often recur (4). It is a common cause of ulcers in the mouth, and secondary infections may occur and cause discomfort. The ulcers are often oval in shape of different sizes and appear single or multiple in otherwise healthy persons. The aetiology is unknown, but suggested causes are vitamin deficiencies, oral microbiota derangements, haematological considerations, stress, and genetic polymorphisms to oxidant-antioxidant imbalances, among others. The therapy is symptomatic and will include pain relief and treatment of secondary infections. Periodic fever, aphthous stomatitis, pharyngitis, and adenitis is an uncommon syndrome in prepubertal children. The fever can occur periodically in a 26-week cycle.

Behçet's disease

In Behçet's disease, oral ulcers appear spontaneously and are one of the diagnostic criteria (5). Although they are not caused primarily by oral infections, the ulcers are exposed to secondary infections by the oral microbiota. The ulcers have a prolonged course before they heal, and this gives rise to much discomfort for the patients. Behçet's disease is of unknown origin, but genetics and immunologic causes have been explored. The prevalence varies in populations. The main symptoms are oral ulcers, genital ulcers, inflammation of the eyes, and arthritis. Complications that may arise are blindness, inflammation of the joints, blood clots, or aneurysm.

Virus, protozoa, candida, and uncommon bacterial infections

Viral infections are known to manipulate the immune system and be the reason for additional opportunistic bacterial infections that may cause oral symptoms. Infection by herpes simplex virus type 1 is common in many populations (6). The primary infection is a general affliction of the oral mucosa, which makes the patient uncomfortable. It lasts 7–10 days. The infection often recurs several times during life and presents by lesions on the lips and skin in the form of blisters in the area supported by the trigeminal cranial nerve. The virus retreats to the trigeminal nerve ganglion and is dormant until a later outbreak of herpetiform ulcerations. Eight different herpes viruses can cause other symptoms, such as genital ulcers, roseola in infants, and possibly Kaposi sarcoma in patients with acquired immunodeficiency syndrome (AIDS).

Varicella-zoster virus is associated with chickenpox as the primary infection and herpes zoster as a secondary infection in adults. The disease presents as a rash with blisters on the skin but may also have oral manifestations.

Epstein–Barr virus is related to mononucleosis and lymphoma. Oral symptoms are leucoplakia and periodontitis, as well as other general symptoms, such as fever and swollen lymph glands. The virus is believed to be associated with later nasopharyngeal carcinoma.

Infection caused by cytomegalovirus is very rare and is associated with periodontitis. Both the Epstein–Barr virus and cytomegalovirus replicate in leukocytes.

Enterovirus is a large group of viruses consisting of five genera – including coxsackievirus and echovirus, which consist of 29 serotypes. Related to oral symptoms are hand, mouth, and foot disease with mouth sores, in addition to other symptoms. It mainly occurs in young children. Herpangina has oral manifestations in the form of blisters on the oral mucosa, ulcerations in the soft palate, and often fever, although it is a rare condition in children of about one week old. Enterovirus illnesses range from mild febrile illness to potentially fatal conditions.

HPV has become a more common infection in the oral cavity in recent years. It has been linked to OSCC, which has been on the increase. HPV is related to cervical cancer in women.

AIDS is caused by the human immunodeficiency virus (HIV) (7, 8). It infects the leucocytes and the CD4+ T-cells. These cells are important in the body's immune defence against microorganisms. Kaposi sarcoma, a defining AIDS condition, can appear on the skin and inside the mouth or in other parts of the body.

The protozoa that have been detected in oral lesions are *Entamoeba gingivalis* and *Trichomonas tenax*.

Candida infection is caused by the fungus *Candida albicans*. It is common in the mouth, nasopharynx, gut, and genital tract and is sometimes a pathogen. It is observed in some infants and may infect the mother. The infection is sometimes seen in patients wearing dentures and patients using catheters. The oral mucous membrane becomes red and swollen, and there may be thick white or cream-coloured areas, and swallowing is uncomfortable. Oral candidiasis is called thrush and can include angular cheilitis at the corner of the mouth. It is also seen as a consequence of immunosuppressive treatment or in patients on antibiotic treatment suppressing bacterial commensals.

Other bacterial infections, such as *Treponema pallidum* causing syphilis, *Mycobacterium tuberculosis* causing tuberculosis, or Gram-negative bacterial infections by *Escherichia coli* or *Pseudomonas aeruginosa*, have been detected in the oral cavities of patients with systemic diseases.

Dermatoses

Dermatoses are conditions of the skin not caused by infections (dermatitis). The conditions mentioned here can also cause oral symptoms or only appear in the mouth.

Lichen planus causes an uncomfortable rash or redness of the oral mucosa with characteristic white stria running across the inflamed areas. The cause is unknown, and only symptomatic treatment can be given.

Exposure to specific pathogenic periodontal bacteria has been found to influence disease activity in patients with systemic lupus erythematosus (SLE) (9). These findings provide a rationale for assessing and improving periodontal health in patients with SLE, in addition to other treatments for SLE.

Several disorders cause blisters in the mouth (10). These are painful when they break down and are immediately subjected to secondary infections by oral bacteria. These include several diseases which are not common disorders: the rare autoimmune blistering diseases – MMP, pemphigus vulgaris, linear IgA disease, epidermolysis bullosa acquisita, and paraneoplastic pemphigus. Erythema multiforme may be mistaken for pemphigus vulgaris in appearance, while oral lichen planus may be indistinguishable from MMP. Angina bullosa haemorrhagica may also present with tense haemorrhagic bullae.

Haematological disorders

Haematological disorders are rare, but a differential diagnosis is by blood test, gingival bleeding, paleness of the oral mucosa, and unusual symptoms in combination with general fatigue. Such observations may arise in children and adults. An observant dentist will refer these patients for further examinations. Such haematological disorders include neutropenias; nonsolid haematological malignancies, including leukaemias and mycloproliferative disorder; solid haematological malignancies, such as non-Hodgkin lymphoma; and haematinic deficiencies.

Gastrointestinal disorders

Inflammatory bowel diseases, including Crohn's disease and ulcerative colitis, not only affect the intestinal tract but may also involve the oral cavity (11). These oral manifestations may assist in the diagnosis and monitoring of disease activity. Indurated tag-like lesions, cobblestoning, and mucogingivitis are the most common specific oral findings encountered in Crohn's disease cases, and aphthous stomatitis and pyostomatitis vegetans are among the nonspecific oral manifestations of inflammatory bowel diseases. With these symptoms, the differential diagnosis should be made, considering side effects of drugs, infections, nutritional deficiencies, and other inflammatory conditions.

Gastro-oesophageal reflux

Reflux of acid from the stomach is not uncommon. It is due to a damaged or weak sphincter muscle in the oesophagus. The acid weakens the tooth enamel and can be seen as erosive lesions on teeth. This may also be observed in patients suffering from bulimia.

Malignancy

Already mentioned are haematological cancers such as nonsolid haematological malignancies (e.g. leukaemias and myeloproliferative disorder) and solid haematological malignancies (e.g. non-Hodgkin's lymphoma). Another type of cancer that may develop oral symptoms is Kaposi sarcoma in AIDS. Kaposi sarcoma develops from the cells that line lymph or blood vessels. It usually appears as tumours on the skin, often dark coloured, or on mucosal surfaces, such as inside the mouth, but can develop in other parts of the body. Kaposi sarcoma is categorized as an epidemic, classic, or endemic.

Hypoplasminogenemia

Hypoplasminogenemia or type 1 plasminogen deficiency is a genetic condition associated with inflamed growths on the mucous membranes. It causes a form of gingivitis triggered by local injury and/or infection. This causes deposition of fibrin and inflammation and may recur after removal. Strict oral plaque control is important.

Pregnancy

Pregnant women may present with gingivitis that may bleed upon tooth brushing in the second and third trimesters. The incidence is less common in the first trimester.

Scurvy

Scurvy or vitamin C (ascorbic acid) deficiency presents with several symptoms. Early symptoms are weakness, feeling tired, and sore arms and legs. These are rather nonspecific symptoms, but additional symptoms, such as bleeding from the gums, changes to hair, and bleeding from the skin, may occur. It is not a very common disease due to the knowledge of its cause and the need for a diet with vitamin C included.

Oral white patches associated with systemic diseases

White patches on the oral mucosa are often difficult to distinguish, as they have several causes. They can be nonadherent and can be wiped off or adherent. Nonadherent can be pseudomembraneous candidosis (thrush), other mycoses, food debris, furred tongue, or drug-associated necrotic debris (for example, aspirin and cocaine).

Adherent can be papillomas (warts – these are rarely of sexual origin), white sponge naevus, geographic tongue (erythema migrans – sometimes associated with type 1 hypersensitivity disorders or psoriasis), frictional keratosis (due to, for example, abnormal orofacial movement), lichen planus, lupus disorders, oral hairy leukoplakia, chronic mucocutaneous candidiasis, or others (for example, the rare dyskeratosis congenita).

Salivary gland

Salivary gland swelling occurs in many systemic diseases, as well as diseases of the salivary glands and may be due to nonmalignant diseases, in addition to cancer.

Sjögren syndrome

Sjögren syndrome is an autoimmune disease that also affects oral health (13, 14). Dryness of the mouth due to decreased production of saliva is the main oral symptom, and xerostomia is a characteristic symptom of Sjögren syndrome. Other characteristic symptoms are salivary gland swelling, ocular dryness, autoantibody production, and increasing mononuclear cell infiltration of the salivary and lacrimal glands. This syndrome may affect 0.2%–3.0% of the population, and most are women, with an estimated ratio of 9:1. The most severe complication of Sjögren syndrome is lymphoma, which may occur in 4%–5% of these patients. It is important to maintain their oral health, as dryness of the mouth causes more caries and PD.

Cancer treatment and drugs

Cytotoxic drugs can cause oral symptoms as used in the treatment of breast cancer and may cause osteonecrosis. Osteonecrosis often manifests in the jaw at an early stage as loss of bone structure being visible on X-rays. Osteonecrosis can be caused by radiation therapy to the jaw. This is a serious consequence, as it may deteriorate oral health with loosening of teeth and increased risk of jaw fracture (12). Patients take different drugs, and a good anamnesis of drug history should be taken to clarify any side effects in the oral cavity and associated structures.

Immediate or late effects of cancer treatment can have severe consequences on oral health. A Norwegian study of 190 children sums this up (15). The highest occurrence of cancer was among the youngest children, 0–6 years. Leukaemia and tumours of the central nervous system were each 30%, lymphomas 12%, and other cancers varied between 1%–7% of the cases. The five-year survival rate was 86%. However, two of three children suffer from the late effects of the disease and/or the treatment. This negatively influences their quality of life. General side effects can be a recurrence of cancer; fatigue; altered psychosocial functions; heart, circulation, or lung disease; reduced cognitive capacity; infertility; and endocrine dysfunction. Specific oral symptoms can be craniofacial growth disturbances, disturbances in tooth development, malocclusion, reduced salivary flow, increased caries prevalence, trismus, and oral mucosal disease. These patients need close follow-up to treat varying symptoms and/or initiate treatment to guide developmental disorders.

Dryness of the mouth induced by a drug can cause an increased risk of caries. Oral contraceptives can cause gingivitis due to the effect of hormones.

Psychofarmaca (e.g. bipolar drugs) cause unwanted grinding and consequent pathological chipping of tooth enamel and excessive loss of tooth substance. Heroin users and other drug abusers have very poor oral health often because of heroin causing sugar craving.

Congenital disorders

There are several but rare disorders that have serious effects on oral health and function. These individuals need special attention and treatment to improve their oral hygiene and dental functionality, and they may need follow-up over many years. These disorders may be inherited, and they affect the development of the jaw and facial bones and, consequently, the functionality of the dentition. Developmental disorders of the teeth become evident late in childhood, and children need a careful follow-up of specialists to maintain optimal dental function for eating, speech, appearance, and quality of life.

Concluding remarks

Several systemic diseases of varying pathology are also the cause of oral health symptoms such as ulcers, sores, swellings, bleeding, and pain. Many such ulcers and sores are prone to secondary infections by oral bacteria, giving much discomfort to individuals. Other symptoms of systemic disease are oral pain, loss of sensation, abnormal facial movements, and oral malodour. Several treatments exist, but such information has not been included in this paper. New treatment options will be available as time passes. Dentists will advise on the best treatment possible and preventive measures for the specific symptoms and conditions. Knowledge is required to achieve and maintain optimal oral health.

References

1.   Porter, SR, Mercadante, V, and Fedele, S. 2017. "Oral Manifestations of Systemic Disease." *British Dental Journal*, No. 223: 683–691.
2.   Farmer and Lawton eds. 1966. *Stones' Oral and Dental Diseases.* 5th ed. Edinburgh: E. & S. Livingstone.

3. Tyldeslcy, WR. 1969. *Oral Diagnosis (Pergamon Press Series on Dentistry, vol. 7, Oxford).*

4. Saikaly, Sami K, Saikaly, Tanya S, Saikaly, Lara E. 2018. "Recurrent Aphthous Ulceration: A Review of Potential Causes and Novel Treatments." *Journal of Dermatological Treatment*, No. 29 (6): 542–552   https://doi.org/10.1080/09546634.2017.1422079

5. Al-Mutawa, SA, and Hegab, SM. 2004. "Behcet's Disease." *Clinical and Experimental Medicine*, No. 4: 103–131. https://doi.org/10.1007/s10238-004-0045-0

6. Grinde, B, and Olsen, I. 2010. "The Role of Viruses in Oral Disease." *Journal of Oral Microbiology*, No. 2: 2127. https://doi.org/10.3402/jom.v2i0.2127

7. Challacombe, SJ. 1991. "Oral Research and Dental Treatment in HIV Infection." *British Dental Journal*, No. 171 (5): 146–148. https://doi.org/10.1038/sj.bdj.4807620

8. Moniaci, D, Greco, D, Flecchia, G, Raiteri, R, and Sinicco, A. 1990. "Epidemiology, Clinical Features and Prognostic Value of HIV-1 Related Oral Lesions." *Journal of Oral Pathology and Medicine*, No. 19 (10): 477–481. https://doi.org/10.1111/j.1600-0714.1990.tb00790.x

9. Bagavant, H, Dunkleberger, ML, Wolska, N, Sroka, M, Rasmussen, A, Adrianto, I, Montgomery, C, Sivils, K, Guthridge, JM, James, JA, Merrill, JT, and Deshmukh, US. 2019. "Antibodies to Periodontogenic Bacteria Are Associated with Higher Disease Activity in Lupus Patients." *Clinical and Experimental Rheumatology*, No. 37 (1): 106–111.

10. Carey, B, and Setterfield, J. 2019. "Mucous Membrane Pemphigoid and Oral Blistering Discases." *Clinical and Experimental Dermatology*, No. 44 (7): 732-739. https://doi.org/10.1111/ced.13996

11. Lankarani, KB, Sivandzadeh, GR, and Hassanpour, S. 2013. "Oral Manifestation in Inflammatory Bowel Disease: A Review." *World Journal of Gastroenterology*, No. 19: 8571–8579. https://doi.org/10.3748/wjg.v19.i46.8571

12. Khan, AA, Morrison, A, Kendler, DL, Rizzoli, R, Hanley DA, Felsenberg, D, McCauley LK, O'Ryan, F, Reid, I, Ruggiero, SL, Taguchi, A, Tetradis, S, Watts, NE, Brandi, ML, Peters, E, Guise, T, Eastell, R, Cheung, MA, Morin, SN, Masri, B, Cooper, C, Morgan, SL, Obermayer-Pietsch, B, Langdahl, BL, AlDabach, R, Davison , KS, Sandor, GK, Josse, RG, Bhandari, M, Rabbani, ME, Pierroz, DD, Sulimani, R, Saunders, DP, Brown, JP, Compston, J, on behalf

of the International Task Force on Osteonecrosis of the Jaw. 2017. "Case-Based Review of Osteonecrosis of the Jaw (ONJ) and Application of the International Recommendations for Management from the International Task Force on ONJ." *Journal of Clinical Densitometry*, No. 20 (1): 8–24. https://doi.org/10.1016/j.jocd.2016.09.005

13.   Reksten, TR, and Jonsson, MV. 2014. "Sjögren's Syndrome: An Update on Epidemiology and Current Insights on Pathophysiology." *Oral and Maxillofacial Surgery Clinics of North America*, No. 26: 1–12. https://doi.org/10.1016/j.coms.2013.09.002

14.   Bolstad, AI, Le Hellard, S, Kristjansdottir, G, Vasaitis, L, Kvarnström, M, Sjöwall, C, Johnsen, SJ, Eriksson, P, Omdal, R, Brun, JG, Wahren-Herlenius, M, Theander, E, Syvänen, AC, Rönnblom, L, Nordmark, G, and Jonsson, R. 2012. "Association between Genetic Variants in the Tumour Necrosis Factor/Lymphotoxin α/Lymphotoxin β Locus and Primary Sjögren's Syndrome in Scandinavian Samples." *Annals of the Rheumatic Diseases*, No. 71: 981–988. https://doi.org/10.1136/annrheumdis-2011-200446

15.   Woicik, DM, Sivertsen, TB, Løes, S, and Midtbø, M. 2021. "Craniofacial and Oral Late Effects after Childhood Cancer Treatment." *Norske Tannlegeforenings Tidende*, No. 131: 454–462.

PART 4:

CARDIOVASCULAR DISEASE RESEARCH

CHAPTER 18

THE OSLO STUDY

Intervention and epidemiology of cardiovascular diseases with interpretation for the benefit of the public health

The epidemiologic knowledge of change and development of predictors for health and disease was explored using the Oslo study of 1972/73. The study was the first population based study in Norway and has been the foundation of much research. In short, a total of 30,025 men in Oslo born in the period 1923–1952, those aged 40–49 years and a 7% sample of men aged 20–39 years, were invited to attend a health screening at Ullevål University Hospital in Oslo, Norway, during the years 1972 and 1973. In all, 17,965 attended the health screening. This was the basic structure from which two randomized controlled trials, as well as epidemiologic prospective analyses of the full cohort were carried out. Over the years and until today, several research questions have been raised and hypotheses tested, and results of these questions and hypotheses have been published. Multiple risk factors, both established and new, have been assessed for their prediction of future health events in this study. References are listed below.

The Oslo study of 1972/73

The principal investigator was Professor Paul Leren, MD, Dr Med. The study is well described. Two intervention trials (RCTs) and prospective cohort follow-up studies on incidence and mortality of CVD were performed. The two intervention trials were on (a) cholesterol reduction and smoking cessation combined compared to no intervention and (b) drug reduction of hypertension compared to placebo effect. (c) The third study analysed risk factors for the development of coronary heart disease. (d) The fourth study used electrocardiogram observations in nonsymptomatic persons. (e) The fifth study approached the association of a long-term follow-up of incidence and mortality of stroke and MI, and the analysis for total mortality was done after 12 and 18 years of follow-up. These studies were all lead to doctoral dissertations, references are listed below. Further follow-up analyses were performed after 21 years regarding the incidence of stroke and MI and after 26 years on air pollution and mortality, as well as metabolic syndrome and prostate cancer. New knowledge of cardiovascular diseases due to the Oslo study of 1972/73 was a major achievement in Norwegian medical research for the benefit of the general public and patients alike.

By 2000, 79 scientific papers and 5 doctoral dissertations had been published based on the Oslo study of 1972/73. Two RCTs had been performed, and long-term follow-up on incidence and mortality of stroke, myocardial infarction, and total mortality had been published.

The Oslo study of 1972/73, considered to be the first population-based study in Norway, was, in many respects, the model and inspiration for future regional population-based studies with the aim of epidemiologic research:

The Tromsø Study started in 1974 because the mortality rate for CVD was high in Northern Norway. The Tromsø Study is the most comprehensive study, and 45,000 men and women have participated in seven repeat surveys. The eighth survey is currently ongoing. In the last survey, oral health was included. https://uit.no/research/tromsostudy

The Trøndelag Health Study (HUNT) started in 1984 and is still a highly active research endeavour, as about 300 national and international research projects use its data. The database includes information for about 230,000 people. https://www.ntnu.edu/hunt

Then the Homocysteine study (1992/1993) and the Hordaland Health Study (1997–1999) population screenings – now collectively termed the Hordaland Health Study (HUSK) – were carried out in West Norway. https://www.uib.no/en/nutrition/111322/husk-hordaland-health-studies

The last major health screening was the Oslo Health Study (HUBRO) in 2001, which included several substudies.
https://www.fhi.no/en/more/health-studies/landsomfattende-helseundersokelser-lhu/helseundersokelser/the-oslo-health-study-hubro/

Major variables from these studies, including the Oslo II-study in 2000, have been assembled in the large database of the Cohort of Norway (CONOR). CONOR contains data of over 200,000 people. From these studies, much research has been performed, giving varied information about disease occurrence and causal pathways of Norwegian women and men, both young and old, for future epidemiologic research. CONOR is included in international cooperation on prospective population-based research. https://www.fhi.no/en/studies/conor/

References of the Oslo study of 1972/73

Description and main results of the screening in 1972/73

a) Leren, P, Askevold, EM, Foss, OP, Froili, A, Grymyr, D, Helgeland, A, Hjermann, I, Holme, I, Lund-Larsen, PG, and Norum, KR. 1975. "The Oslo Study. Cardiovascular Disease in Middle-Aged and Young Men Living in Oslo." *Acta Medica Scandinavica (Supplementum)*, No. 588: 1–38.

Doctoral dissertations

b) Helgeland, A. 1980. "Treatment of mild hypertension: A five-year controlled drug trial." Doctoral dissertation, University of Oslo.

c) Hjermann, I. 1981. "Coronary Heart Disease Prevention." Doctoral dissertation, University of Oslo.

d) Holme, I. 1982. "Coronary Risk Factors and Their Possible Causal Role in the Development of Coronary Heart Disease. The Oslo Study." Doctoral dissertation, University of Oslo.

e) Lund-Larsen, PG. 1994. "ECG in Health and Disease. ECG Findings in Relation to CHD Risk Factors, Constitutional Variables and 16-Year Mortality in 2990 Asymptomatic Oslo Men Aged 40-49 Years in 1972. The Oslo Study." ISM skriftserie nr. 30. Doctoral dissertation, University of Tromsø.

f) Håheim, Lise L. 1998. "Epidemiology of Stroke in Middle-Aged Men. The Oslo Study." Doctoral dissertation, University of Oslo.

Follow-up studies of the Oslo study of 1972/73

g) Håheim, Lise L, Holme, I, Hjermann, I, Leren, P, and Tonstad, Serena. 2004. "Trends in the Incidence of Acute Myocardial Infarction and Stroke: A 21-Year Follow-Up of the Oslo-Study." *Scandinavian Cardiovascular Journal*, No. 38: 21.

h) Håheim, Lise L, Tonstad, S, Hjermann, I, Leren, P, Holme, I. 2007. "Predictivity of Body Mass Index and Other Risk Factors for Fatal Coronary

Heart Disease: A 21-Year Prospective Cohort Study." *Scandinavian Journal of Public Health*, No. 35 (1):4–10. https://doi.org/10.1080/14034940510032293

i) Håheim, Lise L, Holme, Ingar, Hjermann, Ingvar, and Tonstad, Serena. 2006. "Risk-Factor Profile for the Incidence of Subarachnoid and Intracerebral Haemorrhage, Cerebral Infarction, and Unspecified Stroke during 21 Years' Follow-Up in Men." *Scandinavian Journal of Public Health*, No. 34: 589–597.

j) Nafstad, P, Håheim, Lise L, Ofstad, B, Gram, F, Holme, I, Hjermann, I, and Leren, P. 2004. "Urban Air Pollution and Mortality in a Cohort of Norwegian Men." *Environmental Health Perspectives*, No. 112: 610–615.

k) Håheim, Lise L, Wisløff, TF, Holme, I, and Nafstad, P. 2006. "Metabolic Syndrome Predicts Prostate Cancer in a Cohort of Middle Aged Men Followed for 26 Years." *American Journal of Epidemiology*, No. 164: 769–774.

l) Holme, I, Søgaard, AJ, Lund Larsen, PG, Tonstad, S, and Håheim, Lise L. 2006. "Lønner det seg å leve sunt? Resultater fra Oslo-undersøkelser blant de samme menn i 1972/3 og i år 2000. [Is a Healthy Lifestyle Worthwhile?]. *Tidsskr Nor Laegeforen*, No. 126 (17): 2246–2249.

m) Holme, I, Håheim, Lise L, Tonstad, S, and Hjermann, I. 2006. "Effect of Dietary and Antismoking Advice on the Incidence of Myocardial Infarction: A 16-Year Follow-Up of the Oslo Diet and Antismoking Study after Its Close." *Nutrition, Metabolism & Cardiovascular Diseases*, No. 16: 330–338.

n) Ellingsen I, Hjerkinn EM, Arnesen H, Seljeflot I, Hjermann I, and Tonstad S. 2006. Follow-up of diet and cardiovascular risk factors 20 years after cessation of intervention in the Oslo Diet and Antismoking Study. Eur J Clin Nutr, 60(3):378-85. doi: 10.1038/sj.ejcn.1602327.

o) Holme I, Retterstol K, Norum KR, and Hjermann I. 2016. Lifelong benefits on myocardial infarction mortality: 40-year follow-up of the randomized Oslo diet and antismoking study. J Intern Med, 280:221-7

p) Botteri E, de Lange T, Tonstad S, and Berstad P. 2018. Exploring the effect of a lifestyle intervention on cancer risk: 43-year follow-up of the randomized Oslo diet and antismoking study. J Intern Med, 284(3):282-291. doi: 10.1111/joim.12765.

The Oslo II study of 2000

The planning for a large health screening in Oslo called the Oslo Health Study (HUBRO) started in 1998/1999 (1). The aim was to study a wider array of public health issues in a representative sample of Oslo inhabitants. Researchers were invited to add adjoining research projects. A follow-up of the Oslo study of 1972/73 was accepted and carried out as the Oslo II study in 2000 (2, 3). The author of this book, Professor Lise Lund Håheim DDS Dr Philos, was the initiator and principal investigator. The Oslo II study involved a screening carried out from February 17th to June 23rd, 2000. Questionnaire information on several different subjects was collected. Blood pressure, height, weight, and waist circumference were measured. Serum was tested for total cholesterol, triglycerides, HDL cholesterol, and glucose, all in a nonfasting state. Full blood and remaining serum were stored at -80°C for later analyses.

In a small survey, the participants expressed satisfaction with the study, and they received the results of the blood parameters, including supplementary information about their health. The survey identified a few participants with elevated levels of one or more risk factors that needed medical attention. Also included in this screening were questions on oral health not asked in the first survey, including the use of dental services in the last 12 months (e.g. if teeth were extracted and, if so, the number extracted). Four categories of reasons for tooth extractions were given: periodontal disease, caries, orthodontic treatment, and trauma. The participants were also asked if they had other infections of the oral cavity. Some years after the screening, the sera of the men who had attended both health screenings (n = 5,323) were analysed for hs-CRP. The sera of 1,175 participants were also analysed for IgG antibodies to four oral bacteria – namely, Tf, Td, Pg, and Aa (12). The levels of antibodies of known tissue-destructing bacteria in advanced periodontitis indicate an ongoing or past infection. In addition, analyses for Clara cell protein and TNF-α were performed (8). The data has been linked to the national mortality registry (Statistics Norway) for 9.5-, 12.5-, and 17.5-year follow-up. In the 12.5- and 17.5-year follow-up, the incidence of cancer from the National Cancer Registry was included.

In the Oslo II survey in the year 2000, the change in risk factor levels from 1972/1973 was of major interest (2). The results of the repeated measures were reported for SBP, DBP, triglycerides, total cholesterol, glucose, height, weight, smoking habits and amount, and physical activity at leisure and work. Significant differences were observed, with a change in BMI as the most pronounced. Correlation analyses between BMI change and other registered factors were performed to explore factors associated with the observed BMI change among the men (3). These two articles are the papers that fully explain the screening procedures of the Oslo II study. The first is in Norwegian, and the second is in English. Later papers explored hs-CRP for different self-reported conditions at the 9.5-year follow-up and found it to be significantly elevated in specific self-reported health conditions compared to other participants of the cohort (15). Self-reported tooth extractions were further explored (19, 21, 22). In addition, antibodies to the four bacteria and hs-CRP were modelled in statistical analyses (12). The conclusion was that the fourth quartile level to either one of the four antibodies analysed was independent of hs-CRP (HR = 1.30). The specific infection was a stronger predictor than the nonspecific inflammation parameter hs-CRP as a predictor for MI. Hs-CRP has previously been found to be associated with CVD.

Other publications have explored the predictivity of the following oral health indicators:

➢ tooth extraction, alcohol consumption pattern and myocardial infarction (20)
➢ tooth extraction, hs-CRP, diabetes, and mortality (21)
➢ number of tooth extractions and increased risk of mortality (22)
➢ tooth extraction and stroke mortality (23)
➢ antibodies to oral bacteria in periodontal disease associated with mortality of myocardial infarction (24)

Dissertation from the Oslo II study

Madsen, Christian. 2009. "Urban Environmental Exposures and Potential Markers of Risk for Cardiovascular Disease." Doctoral dissertation, University of Oslo.

Master thesis from the Oslo II-study

Lawrence, Graeme. 2020. "Bacteraemia and Cardiovascular Disease. A Case-Cohort Study of the Oslo II Dataset." Master's thesis, Department of Mathematics, Faculty of Mathematics and Natural Sciences, University of Oslo.

References from the Oslo II study

1. https://www.fhi.no/globalassets/dokumenterfiler/studier/helseunder
    sokelsene/hubro-material-and-methods---english-pdf.pdf
2. Håheim, Lise L, Holme, I, Hjermann, I, Søgaard, AJ, Lund Larsen,
    PG, and Leren, P. "Resultater fra Oslo-undersøkelser blant de samme
    menn i 1972/3 og i år 2000. Endring i risikofaktorer for hjerte- og
    karsykdom." [Changes in Cardiovascular Risk Factors among Men
    in Oslo in 28 years]. *Tidsskr Nor Laegeforen*, No. 126 (17): 2240–
    2245.
3. Håheim, Lise L, Lund Larsen, PG, Søgaard, AJ, and Holme, I. 2006.
    "Risk Factors Associated with Body Mass Index Increase in Men at
    28 Years Follow-Up." *QJM*, No. 99 (10): 665–671.
4. Holme, I, Søgaard, AJ, Lund Larsen, PG, Tonstad, S, and Håheim,
    Lise L. 2006. "Lønner det seg å leve sunt? Resultater fra Oslo-
    undersøkelser blant de samme menn i 1972/3 og i år 2000 [Is a
    Healthy Lifestyle Worthwhile?]. *Tidsskr Nor Laegeforen*, No. 126
    (17): 2246–2249.
5. Holme, Ingar, Tonstad, Serena, Søgaard, Anne J, Lund-Larsen, Per
    G, and Håheim, Lise L. 2007. "Leisure Time Physical Activity in
    Middle Age Predicts the Metabolic Syndrome in Old Age: Results
    of a 28-Year Follow-Up of Men in the Oslo Study." *BMC Public
    Health*, No. 7: 154.
6. Holme, Ingar, Søgaard, Anne J, Tonstad, S., Lund-Larsen, Per G,
    and Håheim, Lise L. "Repeated Weight Loss Is Associated with the
    Metabolic Syndrome and Diabetes: Results of a 28 Year Re-
    screening of Men in the Oslo Study." *Metabolic Syndrome and
    Related Disorders*, No. 5: 127–135.
7. Madsen, C, Nafstad, P, Eikvar, L, Schwarze, PE, Ronningen, KS,
    and Håheim, LL. "Association between Tobacco Smoke Exposure
    and Levels of C-reactive Protein in the Oslo II Study." *European
    Journal of Epidemiology*, No. 22 (5): 311–317.
8. Madsen, Christian, Durand, Kevin L, Nafstad, Per, Schwarze, Per E,
    Rønningen, Kjersti S, and Håheim, Lise L. 2008. "Associations
    between Environmental Exposures and Serum Concentrations of
    Clara Cell Protein among Elderly Men in Oslo, Norway."
    Environmental Research, No. 108 (3): 354–360.
9. Søgaard, Anne J, Dalgard, Odd S, Holme, Ingar, Røysamb, Espen,
    and Håheim, Lise L. 2008. "Associations between Type A Behaviour
    Pattern and Psychological Distress. 28 Years of Follow-Up of the
    Oslo Study 1972/73." *Social Psychiatry and Psychiatric Epidemiology*,
    No. 43 (3): 216–223.

10.   Søgaard, Anne J, Meyer, Haakon E, Tonstad, Serena, Håheim, Lise L, and Holme, Ingar. 2008. "Weight Cycling and Risk of Forearm Fractures: A 28-Year Follow-Up of Men in the Oslo Study." *American Journal of Epidemiology*, No. 167 (8): 1005–1013.

11.   Søgaard, Anne J, Meyer, Haakon E, Dalgard, Odd S, Holme, Ingar, and Håheim, Lise L. 2008. "Er det sammenheng mellom psykologisk distress og underarmsbrudd? Osloundersøkelsen 1972/73 og 2000." (Associations between type A behaviour pattern and psychological distress). *Norsk Epidemiologi*, No. 18 (Suppl 1): s. 11-11.

12.   Håheim, Lise L, Olsen, Ingar, Nafstad, Per, Schwarze, Per, and Rønningen, Kjersti S. 2008. "Antibody Levels to Single Bacteria or in Combination Evaluated against Myocardial Infarction." *Journal of Clinical Periodontology*, No. 35: 473–478.

13.   Madsen, Christian, Durand, Kevin L, Nafstad, Per, Schwarze, Per E, Rønningen, Kjersti S, and Håheim, Lise L. "Associations between Environmental Exposures and Serum Concentrations of Clara Cell Protein among Elderly Men in Oslo, Norway." *Environmental Research*, No. 108: 354–360.

14.   Håheim, Lise L, Olsen, Ingar, Nafstad, Per, Schwarze, Per, and Rønningen, Kjersti S. 2008. "Ikke enkeltbakterier, men et knippe av bakterier øker risikoen for myokardinfarkt." (C-reactive protein variations for different chronic somatic disorders). *Norske Tannlegeforenings Tidende*, No. 10: 664.

15.   Håheim, Lise L, Olsen, Ingar, Nafstad, Per, Schwarze, Per, and Rønningen, Kjersti S. 2009. "C-reactive Protein Variations for Different Chronic Somatic Disorders." *Scandinavian Journal of Public Health*, No. 37 (6): 640–646.

16.   Søgaard, Anne J, Meyer, Haakon E; Dalgard, Odd S, Holme, Ingar, and Håheim, Lise L. 2009. "Psychological Distress and Forearm Fracture in Men. The Oslo Study 1972/73 and 2000." *Osteoporosis International*, No. 20 (Suppl 4) s. 310.

17.   Håheim, Lise L, Olsen, Ingar, and Rønningen, Kjersti S. 2010. "Regular Alcohol Consumption, Oral Infection Status, and the Association to Myocardial Infarction." *European Heart Journal*, No. 31: 813.

18.   Håheim, Lise L, Nafstad, Per, Olsen, Ingar, Schwarze, Per, and Rønningen, Kjersti S. 2010. "C-reaktivt protein (CRP) varierer ved forskjellige kroniske lidelser." *Norske Tannlegeforenings Tidende*, No. 120: 46.

19.   Håheim, LL, Olsen, I, and Rønningen, KS. 2011. "Association between Tooth Extraction and Myocardial Infarction." *Community Dentistry and Oral Epidemiology*, No. 39 (5): 393–397.

20.   Håheim, Lise L, Olsen, I, and Rønningen, KS. 2012. "Oral Infection, Regular Alcohol Drinking Pattern and Myocardial Infarction." *Medical Hypothesis*, No. 79 (6): 725–730.

21.   Håheim, Lise L, Rønningen, KS, Enersen, M, and Olsen, I. 2017. "The Predictive Role of Tooth Extractions, Oral Infections, and hs-C-reactive Protein for Mortality in Individuals with and without Diabetes: A Prospective Cohort Study of a 12 1/2-Year Follow-Up." *Journal of Diabetes Research*, No. 2017: 9590740. https://doi.org/10.1155/2017/9590740

22.   Håheim, Lise L, Rønningen, KS, Nafstad, P, Schwarze, PE, Thelle, DS, and Olsen, I. 2017. "Number of Tooth Extractions Is Associated with Increased Risk of Mortality." *SciTz Dentistry: Research & Therapy*, No. 2 (1).

23.   Håheim, Lise L, Nafstad, Per, Schwarze, Per E, Olsen, Ingar, Rønningen, Kjersti S, and Thelle, Dag S. 2019. "Oral Health and Cardiovascular Disease Risk Factors and Mortality of Cerebral Haemorrhage, Cerebral Infarction and Unspecified Stroke in Elderly Men: A Prospective Cohort Study." *Scandinavian Journal of Public Health*, No. 48: 762–769. https://doi.org/10.1177/1403494819879351

24.   Håheim, Lise L, Schwarze, PE, Thelle, DS, Nafstad, P, Rønningen, KS, and Olsen, I. 2020. "Low Levels of Antibodies for the Oral Bacterium *Tannerella forsythia* Predict Cardiovascular Disease Mortality in Men with Myocardial Infarction: A Prospective Cohort Study." *Medical Hypotheses*, No. 138: 109575. https://doi.org/10.1016/j.mehy.2020.109575

International cooperation

Oslo II results have been presented at several conferences nationally and internationally. Specific data elements have been included in the meta-database of Norwegian regional cohort studies – CONOR, which is administered by the Norwegian Institute for Public Health. The Oslo study of 1972/73 and the Oslo II study (separate) are both part of two international collaborations on cohort studies on cardiovascular diseases: Prospective Studies Collaboration, administered by the University of Oxford, England, and Emerging Risk Factors Collaboration, administered by Cambridge University, England.

References from international meta-cohort studies

1. Prospective Studies Collaboration. 1995. "Cholesterol, Diastolic Blood Pressure, and Stroke: 13,000 Strokes in 450,000 People in 45 Prospective Cohorts." *Lancet*, No. 346: 1647–1653.
2. Prospective Studies Collaboration. 1999. "Collaborative Overview ("Meta-analysis") of Prospective Observational Studies of the Associations of Usual Blood Pressure and Usual Cholesterol Levels with Common Causes of Death: Protocol for the Second Cycle of the Prospective Studies Collaboration." *Journal of Cardiovascular Risk*, No. 6: 315–320.
3. Prospective Studies Collaboration. 2002. "Age-Specific Relevance of Usual Blood Pressure to Vascular Mortality: One Million Adults in 61 Prospective Cohorts." *Lancet*, No. 360: 1903–1913.
4. Prospective Studies Collaboration. Whitlock, G, Lewington, S, Sherliker, P, Clarke, R, Emberson, J, Halsey, J, Qizilbash, N, Collins, R, and Peto, R. 2009. "Body-Mass Index and Cause-Specific Mortality in 900 000 Adults: Collaborative Analyses of 57 Prospective Studies." *Lancet*, No. 373 (9669): 1083–1096.
5. Prospective Studies Collaboration and Asia Pacific Cohort Studies Collaboration. 2018. "Sex-Specific Relevance of Diabetes to Occlusive Vascular and Other Mortality: A Collaborative Meta-analysis of Individual Data from 980 793 Adults from 68 Prospective Studies." *Lancet Diabetes & Endocrinology*, No. 6 (7): 538–546.
6. Emerging Risk Factors Collaboration. 2014. "Glycated Hemoglobin Measurement and Prediction of Cardiovascular Disease." *JAMA*, No. 311 (12): 1225–1233.
7. Emerging Risk Factors Collaboration. 2015. "Association of Cardiometabolic Multimorbidity with Mortality." *JAMA*, No. 314 (1): 52–60.
8. Emerging Risk Factors Collaboration. 2019. "Equalization of four Cardiovascular Risk Algorithms after Systematic Recalibration: Individual-Participant Meta-analysis of 86 Prospective Studies." *European Heart Journal*, No. 40 (7): 621–631.
9. Emerging Risk Factors Collaboration. 2019. "Cardiovascular Risk Factors Associated with Venous Thromboembolism." *JAMA Cardiology*, No. 4 (2): 163–173.

Concluding remarks

It has been a tremendous research journey for me to be part of the Oslo Study 1972/73 from the late 1980s until now. There are a great number of people and many institutions to thank for advancing this research endeavour. It required a great deal of work by several people. We have all learned so much and brought important information to the research community with the aim of improving public health.